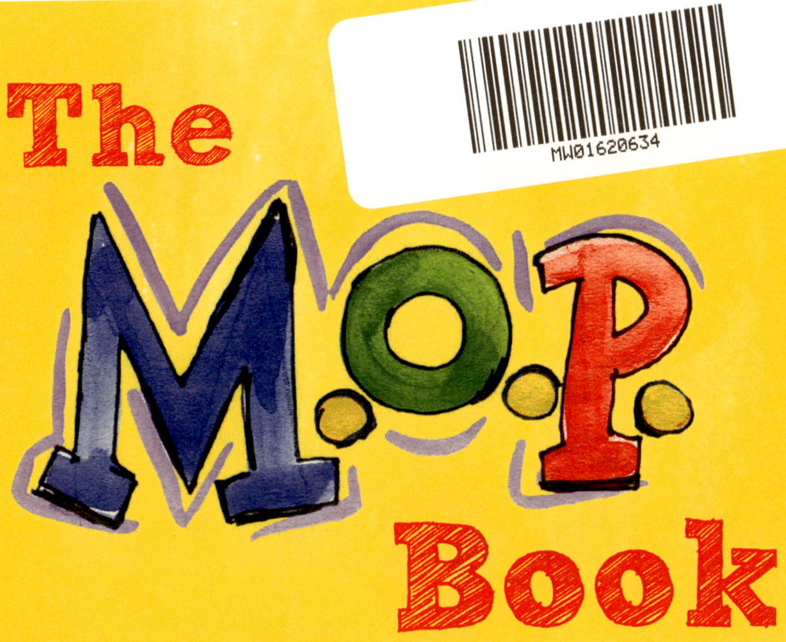

The M.O.P. Book

A Guide to the Only Proven Way to STOP Bedwetting and Accidents

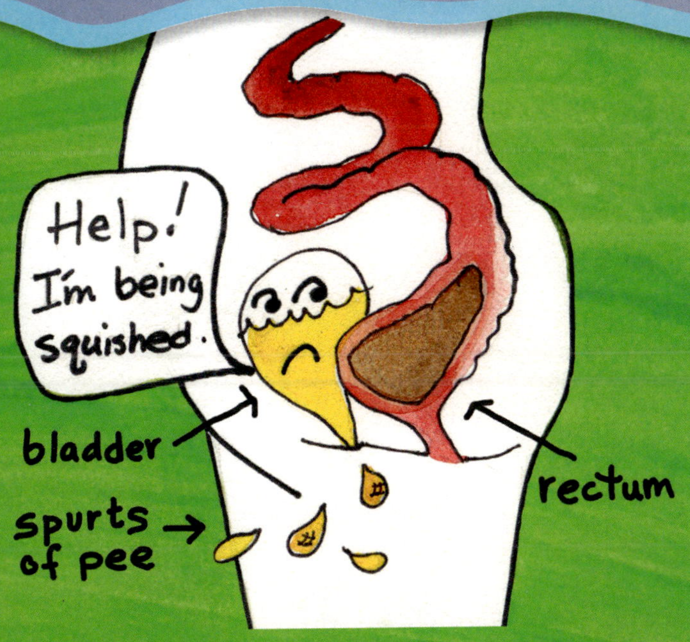

By Steve Hodges, M.D., with Suzanne Schlosberg
Illustrations by Cristina Acosta

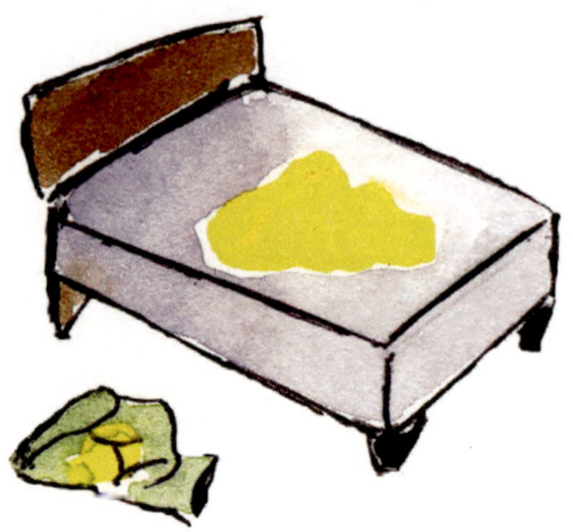

BedwettingAndAccidents.com

The M.O.P. Book

Book design: DyanRothDesign.com

O'Regan Press

Library of Congress Cataloging-in-Publication Data is available on file.

Softcover: 978-0-9908774-3-1
eBook: 978-0-9908774-4-8

Printed in Canada

The M.O.P. Book

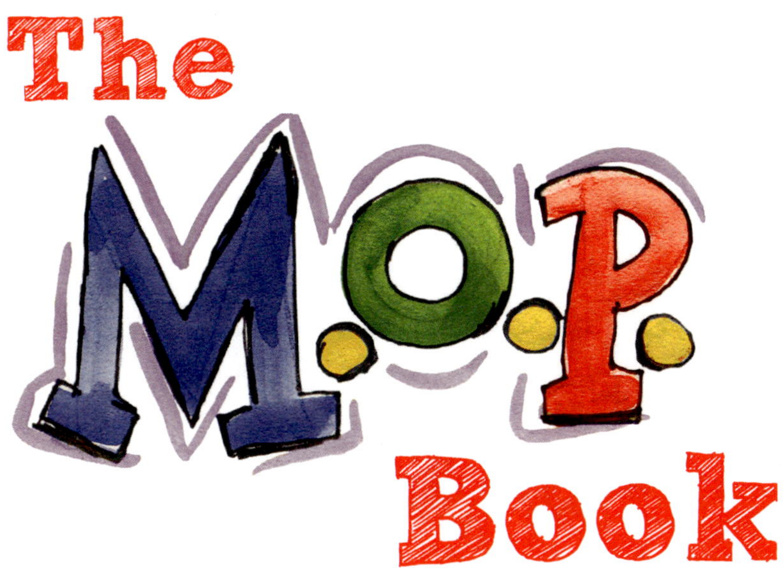

A Guide to the Only Proven Way to STOP Bedwetting and Accidents

By Steve Hodges, M.D., with Suzanne Schlosberg
Illustrations by Cristina Acosta

Contents

PART 1

INTRODUCING M.O.P.

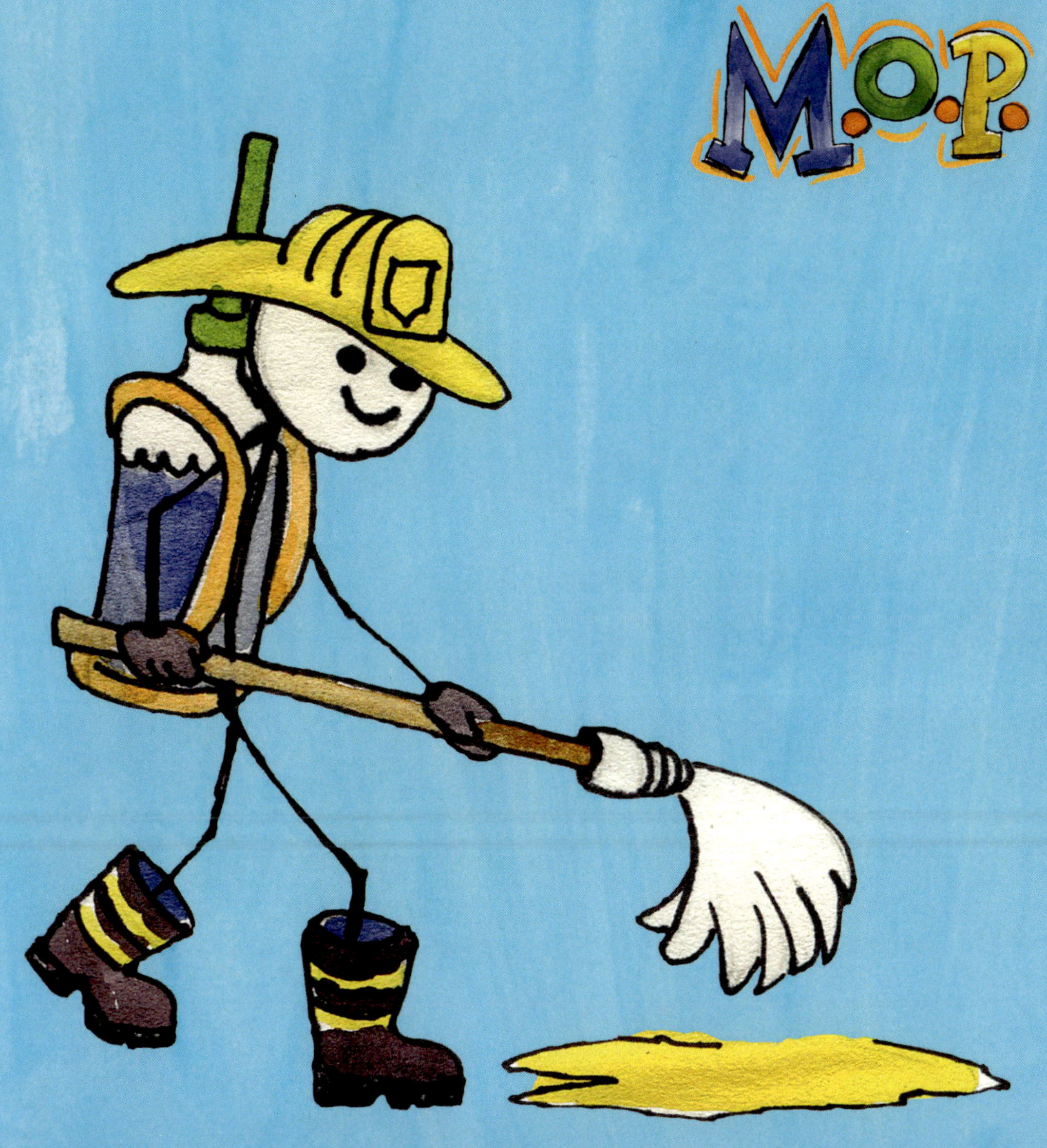

PART 1:
INTRODUCING M.O.P.

Have you been told your child is sure to "outgrow" bedwetting? That accidents are normal? Or that bedwetting is caused by a "small bladder," "deep sleep," stress, or behavior issues?

None of that is true!

Bedwetting and accidents are incredibly common — epidemic, I would argue — but they are not normal, and they are totally fixable. Fact is, more than 90% of accidents — daytime and nighttime, pee and poop — are caused by a chronic pile-up of stool in the rectum. Yes, constipation.

In this part, I explain how constipation triggers bedwetting and accidents, and I introduce **M.O.P.**, the only reliable fix for stressful problems.

What the Heck Is M.O.P.?

OK, folks, quick question: If your bathtub drain pipe was clogged with hair, would you wait around for the pipe to unclog itself?

Of course not, because patience does not unclog drains!

Patience generally doesn't solve bedwetting and accidents, either. And yet the prevailing remedy for childhood toileting problems is simply to hang tight. "Don't even worry about it until she's 7," doctors routinely tell parents. Or: "Eventually he'll grow out of it — nobody goes to college wetting the bed."

That's not helpful! Plus, it's not even true. I have my share of teenage patients whose bedwetting was dismissed for more than a decade. Their biggest fear is heading off to college with pull-ups.

Potty accidents may not be life-threatening, but they can be demoralizing, embarrassing, and exhausting. Not to mention, pull-ups aren't cheap. When a child has chronic accidents, the whole family suffers. I see it all the time: Parents are judged, and kids are teased and blamed. I often write notes on behalf of students threatened with suspension for accidents at school.

The Modified O'Regan Protocol is appropriate for:

- Children age 4+ who wet the bed
- Toilet-trained children who have daytime pee accidents and/or poop accidents
- Toilet-trained girls who have recurrent urinary tract infections

And yet families are advised to wait it out. Or, they're offered useless, even harmful advice, like "offer rewards on dry nights" or "have her drink less fluid and practice holding her pee during the day." Most often, they're offered inadequate treatments, such as bladder medication, bedwetting alarms, or a daily dose of MiraLAX.

All these treatments fall short because they don't address the actual cause of bedwetting and accidents: chronic, severe constipation.

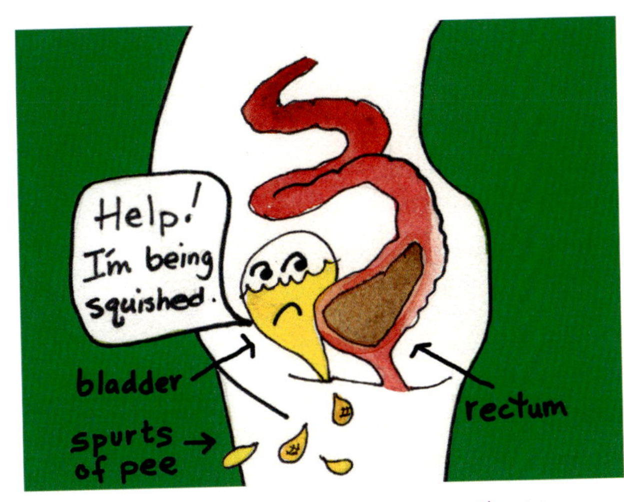

The mass of poop presses against the bladder.

How does constipation cause accidents?

Well, when a child regularly withholds poop — a problem rampant in Western culture — stool piles up in the rectum, forming a large, hard mass. The rectum stretches to accommodate this mass lump (think: rat in a snake's belly), squishing and irritating the bladder. The consequences can be messy:

- **Bedwetting (nocturnal enuresis):** Squished and irritated, the bladder can't hold enough pee overnight.
- **Daytime pee accidents (enuresis):** The irritated bladder hiccups and empties without warning.
- **Poop accidents (encopresis):** The stretched rectum loses tone and sensation, so poop drops out of the child's bottom, often without the child even noticing.
- **Chronic UTIs (in girls):** The child harbors extra infection-causing bacteria in the rectum, too close to the outside world. These bacteria colonize the area between the vagina and anus and eventually the bladder.

All these conditions can be resolved! The remedy is to clean out the clogged rectum and keep it clear on a daily basis. Only then can the rectum shrink back to size, stop bothering the bladder, and regain tone and sensation.

But here's the catch: You need to treat the constipation aggressively. Most doctors don't. Even those aware of the bedwetting-constipation link tend to undertreat the rectal clog, prescribing a daily dose of oral laxative. That's like cleaning a food-encrusted dinner plate with a trickle of water. Totally ineffective!

I know, because I used to be one of those doctors prescribing inadequate treatments. I didn't grasp how constipated these kids are, and I was just following what I'd been taught in medical school. I figured bedwetting just wasn't very treatable.

But I was wrong. A decade later, I know what works: a daily enema regimen I call **M.O.P.**, short for the Modified O'Regan Protocol. **M.O.P.** is named for Sean O'Regan, M.D., the pediatric kidney specialist who pioneered this approach back in the 1980s and published studies showing it's remarkably effective.

Based on my experience with Dr. O'Regan's protocol and my own published research, I've modified his regimen slightly. But the crux of the treatment — daily enemas for a month, followed by tapering — was Dr. O'Regan's idea.

To folks unfamiliar with **M.O.P.**, it sounds nuts — I know! Your doctor's eyes might bug out when you mention "daily enemas." But that just means the physician has no experience with **M.O.P.**, hasn't read the supporting research, or both.

Don't accept claims that daily enemas are "too aggressive" or "too invasive" or "traumatic for children." **M.O.P.** is none of those things. (Know what's traumatic? Wetting the bed in high school.)

Still, I understand enemas are nobody's idea of family fun. If you are reluctant to give your child daily enemas — if you worry about hurting, endangering, or embarrassing your child — you have plenty of company. I understand these concerns! In this guide, I discuss the research behind **M.O.P.**, how to implement the protocol, and how to gain your child's buy-in.

You may not get the resistance you expect, as children are more distraught about their toileting problems than they let on. Robin Lund, DPT, a South Dakota physical therapist who specializes in childhood incontinence and recommends **M.O.P.**, tells me her patients often hide the true extent of their distress. "I have had many children admit to me with tears in their eyes that it bothers them to have accidents, even though they have told their parents the opposite," says Robin.

When you explain to these kids that enemas will make the accidents stop, they're usually willing, even eager, to go along.

Not long ago I received an email from the mom of a 5-year-old who was having both daytime and nighttime accidents. Their pediatrician advised against enemas, but when MiraLAX clean-outs failed, the family moved forward with **M.O.P.**

At first her daughter was fearful and found the enemas uncomfortable. But it wasn't long before the process became routine. "Now my daughter sings 'I just can't wait for my enema' to the Lion King song!" her mom wrote.

Her symptoms — and confidence — have improved dramatically. "Her entire demeanor has changed after 36 days on **M.O.P.**," her mom reported. "She's a happy kid again. She doesn't come home from school wet, she doesn't fear the pee smell, and best yet, she's been dry at night. She was soaking her whole life, so this is huge."

As you embark on M.O.P., keep in mind that this protocol is not a magic cure but a process that involves trial and error. Although most of my patients experience major progress, if not total dryness, within the first 30 days, some do not. In these cases, the families need to change aspects of the regimen as they move forward. Prepare your family for this possibility, and know that there is always a next step to try.

I am always learning from my patients' experiences, and I welcome feedback from all who try **M.O.P.**

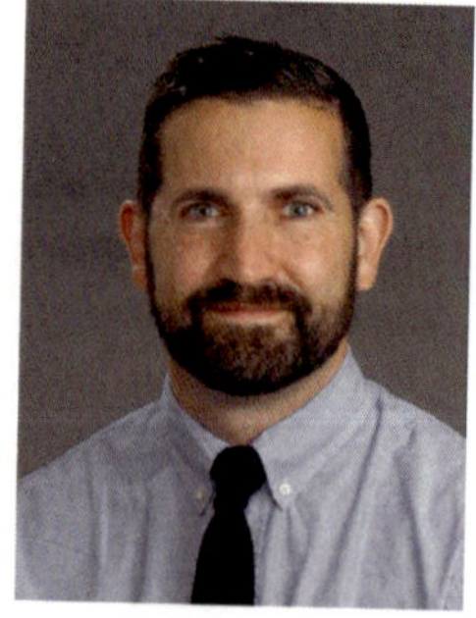

Steve Hodges, M.D.

Associate Professor of Pediatric Urology,
Wake Forest University School of Medicine

M.O.P. in a Nutshell

1) Do daily enemas for at least 30 days.

Taper only when the child remains accident-free for at least 5 consecutive days. If the child has no dry days or nights in the first month, switch to M.O.P.+

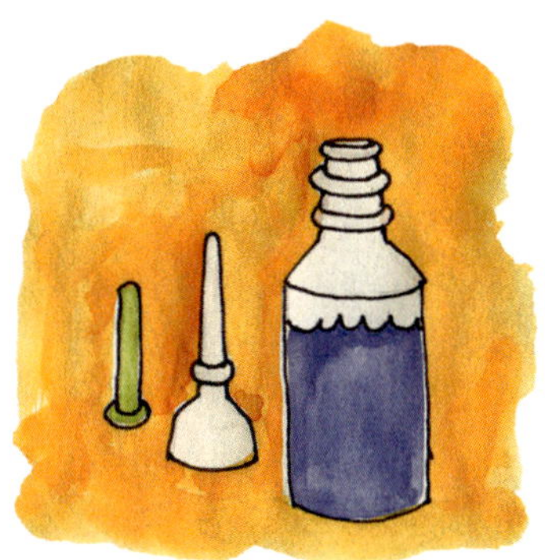

2) After at least 30 days of enemas and five consecutive days of dryness, taper to one enema every other day for another 30 days.

If accidents recur, resume daily enemas until achieving 5 consecutive accident-free days.

3) After a second 30 days of dryness, taper to enemas twice a week for 30 days before stopping.

If accidents recur, resume daily enemas until 5 consecutive accident-free days, and then taper to every other day for 30 days.

4) Take an osmotic laxative daily to keep poop mushy.

Use MiraLAX, lactulose, or other laxative of your choice. Take a full dose daily or half a dose twice a day. Continue daily laxatives throughout M.O.P. and for 3 to 6 months afterward.

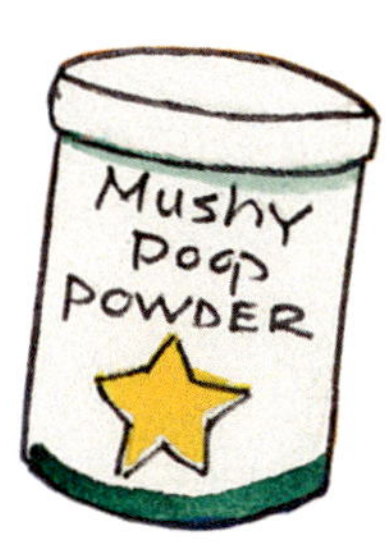

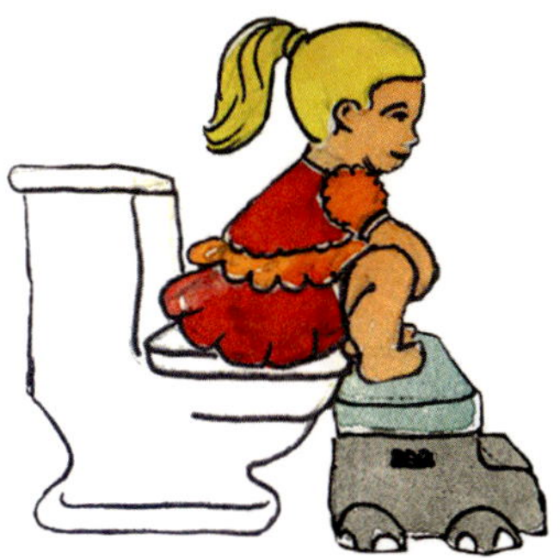

5) Poop with feet on a stool.

The stool must be tall enough to place the child in a squatting position. Small children should sit on a child-sized toilet seat to help the pooping muscles relax.

What to Expect from M.O.P.

The first question I usually get from parents is: How long will it take for the accidents to stop?

The short answer: anywhere from a few weeks to several months, depending on your child's symptoms and physiology. I wish it could happen faster! But a rectum clogged for years won't rebound overnight. Also, when the nerves feeding the bladder have been chronically irritated, it can take months for them to settle down, even after the rectum is persistently clear.

In some ways, overcoming accidents is like learning to read: a process that happens in fits and starts and that each child experiences differently. Expect uneven progress and setbacks. Occasionally, accidents even increase at first. That's because the volume of enema solution stretches the colon even further and, for unknown reasons, does not stimulate a complete evacuation of stool. So there's even more pressure on the bladder. This scenario is unusual and always temporary.

Though I can't predict how long it will take for your child to achieve dryness, I can offer general observations based on my experience.

Before accidents diminish, your child will experience subtle signs of progress, such as:

- **fewer stomachaches**
- **less frequent need to pee**
- **less urgency to pee**
- **fewer underwear skid marks**
- **improved ability to sense the urge to poop**
- **more spontaneous pooping (other than after an enema)**

Then you should notice more dramatic improvements. If your child does not make progress within 30 days of trying something new — whether starting **M.O.P.** or **M.O.P.+** or using a new enema ingredient — it is important to make a change in your regimen.

Finally, no matter how good your initial results, finish out the protocol as described. Quitting enemas early greatly increases the odds of relapse. Some families even choose to complete two months of every-other-day enemas before tapering to twice a week. When a child has been having accidents for years, I think this is a wise choice.

We tend to see improvement in the following order:
Poop accidents diminish
then STOP
Daytime pee accidents diminish
then STOP
Overnight accidents diminish
then STOP

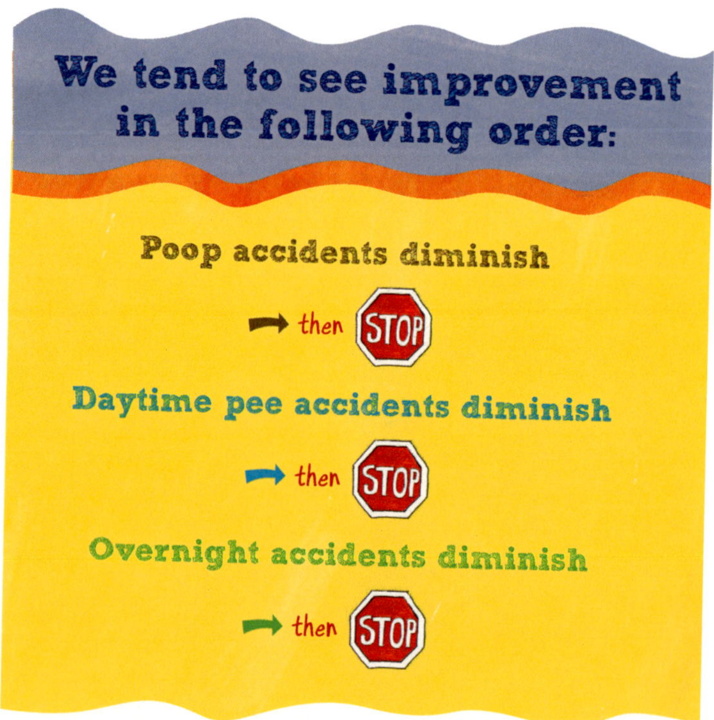

Here's more detail about what to expect based on your child's symptoms.

Poop accidents: These often stop within a week or two on **M.O.P.** These kids are so monumentally clogged that even small improvements make a big difference. Nearly all encopresis cases completely resolve within a month. Still, to prevent a relapse, it's important to finish the 90-day program.

Daytime pee accidents: My research shows 85% of children with daytime pee accidents will stop daytime wetting within 90 days on **M.O.P.** (The remaining 15% need **M.O.P.+**, the large-volume enema protocol.) Most children on **M.O.P.** who have both daytime and nighttime wetting will at least stop having daytime accidents within the first month. It will likely take longer for their bedwetting to cease.

Bedwetting: In my practice, about 95% of bedwetting-only patients see significant progress within 30 days on **M.O.P.**, and around 80% achieve dryness in the first month. But for some children — especially those who have both daytime and nighttime wetting — bedwetting can take several months to resolve. In general, the longer the child has been wetting the bed, the longer it takes for the wetting to stop.

What if your child sees no progress after 30 days? That's when you get an X-ray (see Part 3) and switch to **M.O.P.+** (see Part 6).

Gaining Your Child's Buy-in

"No way will my child agree to enemas!"

I hear that every day, and as a parent, I get it. But I also know most kids will come around if approached in a way that respects their intelligence and feelings and perhaps includes a dash of humor. Your child may actually be less squeamish about enemas than you are! So try not project your own fears onto your child.

Before long, enemas become routine for all involved. Some kids feel so much better after emptying each night that they actually remind Mom or Dad that it's time for the enema.

Here are some ideas to get your child on board.

- **Offer a reward.** Many parents allow their child to play with an iPad or smartphone throughout the process. Others offer a small toy for the first couple days and/or a larger prize after 30 days.
- **Build up to it.** You'll have a revolt on your hands if you bust open the enema package and announce, "Here's what we're doing today!" But you may have success by gently opening a discussion and providing details over a period of days.
- **Give yourself an enema first. Yes, you!** What better way to show empathy and offer a scouting report? Children greatly app reciate this gesture.
- **Read *Bedwetting and Accidents Aren't Your Fault* with your child.** Children will learn that they are not alone — lots of kids have accidents and do enemas. Our book explains how enemas help and what's involved, and our fun illustrations are likely to generate a few laughs.

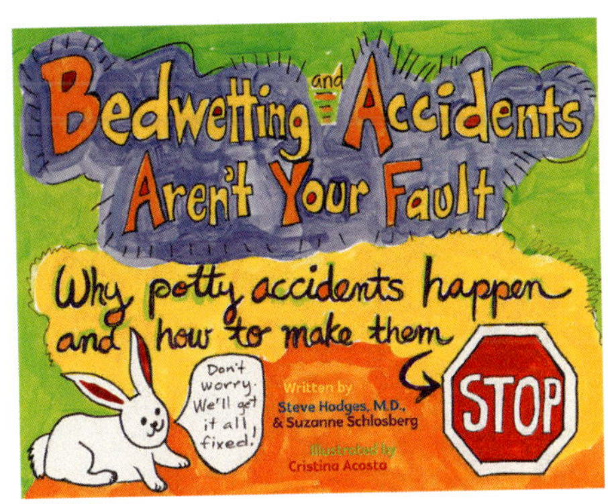

Our children's book makes kids feel better.

Advice from the Trenches

Mom of a 6-year-old

"During the enema, my son distracts himself watching YouTube on my phone. He might flinch because it feels weird but doesn't complain of pain."

Mom of a 4-year-old

"At first we used a sticker chart and my son earned little toys. But after a week we didn't even need the chart."

15-year-old girl

"I was ready to try anything that might end my bedwetting. I learned very quickly how to give myself the enemas, and there is no discomfort at all. I give it to myself on my hands and knees and then lay on my left side on the floor for 5 minutes."

Mom of a 9-year-old

"To ease the weirdness, we laughed about the silliness of the position, with her lying on her side and holding her knees to her chest. My best advice is try to stay mellow so your unease doesn't rub off on your child."

Mom of a 12-year-old

"I try to keep everything very lighthearted. We make inappropriate bum jokes. We've laughed about imagining other kids he knows in the same situation... We've established a ritual around it. He is covered in a blanket as much as possible – I respect his privacy. He takes a bath when he's done, and I think it's become a calming way to end the day."

Physical Therapy for the Pooping and Peeing Muscles

If you've ever torn a hamstring tendon or blown out a knee, you know physical therapy (PT) is an important part of the recovery process. But did you know physical therapy also can help children who have toileting difficulties?

In many chronically constipated children, the muscles that control peeing and pooping — known as the "pelvic-floor" muscles — don't work as they're supposed to. The specialists trained to help children regain coordination in these muscles are called pelvic-floor physical therapists. These experts have much to offer children who are working to overcome bedwetting and accidents, helping speed recovery and prevent relapse.

How exactly does pelvic-floor PT fit in with **M.O.P.**?

Well, fully emptying poop requires three things: 1.) a powerful colon and rectal contraction, 2.) soft poop, and 3.) relaxed pooping muscles. **M.O.P.** helps with the first two; PT targets number three.

Below I have invited two of the country's most experienced pelvic-floor physical therapists, Erin Wetjen, PT, and Robin Lund, DPT., to briefly explain how PT can help chronically constipated children. Erin is the physical therapist for the pediatric urology department at Mayo Clinic in Rochester, Minnesota, and Robin is a pediatric incontinence specialist in Sioux Falls, South Dakota.

Q: **Among children with chronic constipation, what exactly goes wrong with the toileting muscles?**

A: **Instead of relaxing their pelvic muscles when they poop, many of these children tense up — an understandable reaction, given their history of large, painful bowel movements.** Some kids keep their pelvic-floor muscles tightened all day long. Having these muscles constantly "on guard" only worsens their difficulties.

Eventually, all this holding inhibits the natural reflex to pee or poop, and these kids may not even feel the urge. What's more, the pelvic-floor muscles fatigue, like an overstretched rubber band that has lost its elasticity, and poop just falls out or pee leaks out during activities such as playing or jumping.

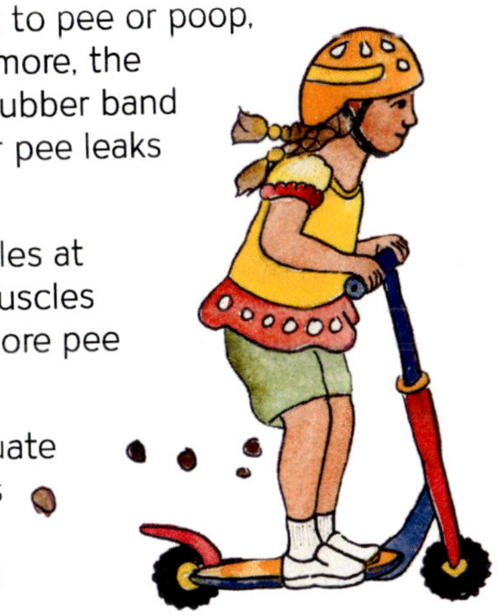

Interestingly, some children not only contract muscles at times they should be relaxed, but they also relax muscles when they should be contracted, like when they store pee and poop until it's time to empty.

We use a tool called "surface biofeedback" to evaluate a child's ability to relax and contract these muscles at the appropriate times. The therapist places small sensors on either side of the child's anus and instructs the child to squeeze or relax. Viewing a computer screen with customized images — dolphins jumping and diving or flowers opening and closing, for example — the child and caregivers are able to see how much these muscles are squeezing and relaxing. Biofeedback also helps the child understand what their muscles feel like when they are contracting and relaxing.

When pooping muscles are fatigued, poop can drop out.

Q: What other services do pelvic-floor PTs offer constipated children, besides helping them retrain their toileting muscles?

A: We provide a comprehensive evaluation and treatment plan, educating families on several fronts, including:

- **Proper toilet posture and positioning** for complete bowel and bladder emptying
- **Sensory training** to respond appropriately to the urges to pee and poop
- **Strategies for the school setting** and dealing with social challenges related to leakage
- **Setting a toileting schedule**
- **Proper hygiene techniques**
- **Breathing patterns while peeing and pooping**
- **Exercises to do at home**
- **Dietary recommendations**

Our patients have a wide variety of symptoms, including enuresis (daytime and nighttime), encopresis, recurrent urinary tract infections, urinary urgency and frequency, urinary retention, and vesicoureteral reflux (backward flow of urine from the bladder into the kidneys). Whatever their symptoms, our goal is to give children a sense of control and confidence while they work toward resolving their conditions.

Q: For children who have continence issues, at what age do you recommend starting pelvic-floor physical therapy?

A: We find that depending on the child's symptoms and maturity level, PT can help starting at age 4 or 5. We treat children up to 18 years of age.

Q: What does pelvic-floor physical therapy involve?

A: After an initial evaluation, the therapist will develop a customized treatment plan. Appointments typically last 30 to 60 minutes. Treatment typically requires six to eight visits over the course of several weeks or months, but plans vary based on the child's progress and severity of the issues.

Q: Where can I find a qualified pelvic-floor physical therapist?

A: The Find a Provider list at BedwettingAndAccidents.com includes PTs who specialize in treating children and are aware of M.O.P. You can also get PT referrals from your pediatrician, pediatric urologist, pediatric gastroenterologist, or the PT department at a local children's hospital. Another option is to contact a local physical therapy clinic and ask if they have, or know of, a pelvic-floor PT experienced in working with children.

> "Our daughter Heidi has struggled with constipation and wetting accidents since she was a toddler. Biofeedback has helped her gain bladder sensation awareness and, more importantly, confidence."
> – Mom of a 9-year-old

Why Bedwetting Drugs Fail

In my clinic I recently saw a teenage patient who'd never had a dry night — despite having spent two years on desmopressin, a medication that suppresses urine production and was prescribed to him by another urologist.

His mom asked, "Do you think he should stay on the medication?"

Desmopressin has a pathetic success rate. Only about one-third of patients who take this drug achieve dryness for 14 days straight — and among those kids, two-thirds relapse when they stop taking the drug. So at best, 11% of kids achieve any kind of "sustained" dryness. (How are they six months later? Nobody has checked.)

Yet desmopressin is considered by major medical organizations to be a "first line" treatment for bedwetting. I am amazed at my profession's enthusiasm for such an ineffective drug.

Consider: In an article titled "Practical consensus guidelines for the management of enuresis," a group of urologists concluded that since desmopressin is effective only on the night it's taken, "therefore, it must be taken on a daily basis." If wetting resumes once the child stops taking the drug, according to the researchers, desmopressin "should be continued/resumed." In other words: If the drug isn't working, keep taking it!

It may be worth noting that four of the six authors of that "consensus guideline" have been involved in drug trials sponsored by companies that manufacture desmopressin.

By the time patients are referred to me, most have been placed on at least one medication for bedwetting. If it's not desmopressin, it's one of the anticholinergics, bladder-relaxing drugs that have a dismal success rate and — get this — commonly cause constipation! Less common side-effects include, in the words of Canadian researchers, "disturbing adverse effects" such as hallucinations, agitation, sedation, confusion, amnesia, and nightmares.[1]

But that doesn't stop many urologists from prescribing these drugs, often in conjunction with desmopressin! Doctors compensate for the constipation by prescribing MiraLAX, so now you've got kids taking three drugs and still wetting the bed.

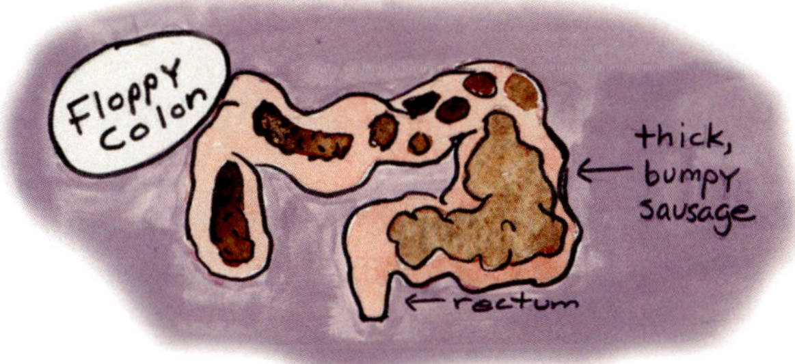

Bedwetting drugs do nothing to address the actual cause of bedwetting: a stretched rectum.

This is nuts. Sure, I understand the appeal of medication — writing a prescription is easy for a doctor and can reassure distressed parents something is being done. But bedwetting is not a disease, like type 1 diabetes, that needs to be controlled with daily medication. It is a condition that can be fixed — permanently — by cleaning out a child's clogged rectum and letting it shrink back to size.

Nonetheless, researchers are on a mission to find the magic drug that will keep kids dry. They are so desperate in their search that even when a drug is shown to be an utter failure, they deem it worthy of consideration. For example, when Swedish researchers tested reboxetine, an antidepressant, on bedwetting patients and only one child — one!

1 Bat-Chen Friedman, MD, et al. Oxybutynin for treatment of nocturnal enuresis in children. Can Fam Physician. 2011 May; 57(5): 559–561.

— out of 18 achieved dryness, the researchers proclaimed the drug "an evidence-based alternative" in the treatment of bedwetting.[2] They even speculated that the low success rate "may be due to the low dosage used." Here's an alternative theory: Maybe antidepressants are simply not effective in treating bedwetting!

The drugs commonly prescribed by urologists don't fix the problem; they just cover it up. Of course, Band-Aids have their place, which is why, on occasion and purely as a stop-gap measure for sleep-away camp or a class trip, I will prescribe medication. But there is no sound rationale for prescribing desmopressin on an ongoing basis, as this drug addresses a problem — urine overproduction — that does not exist.

Desmopressin mimics antidiuretic hormone (ADH), which regulates fluid levels, essentially tricking the kidneys into producing less urine at night. But wait: Do children who wet the bed have abnormal hormone levels? That's a good question to ask a doctor who wants to put your child on this drug. The answer is almost always no.

Though desmopressin is generally safe, the idea of altering the hormones that control urine output in children doesn't sit well with me. If a child is producing plenty of urine at night and is otherwise healthy, there is probably a good reason the child's body is producing that pee. We all need to get rid of fluid to maintain our body's fluid and electrolyte balance, so why mess with that? Especially since desmopressin does nothing to resolve the constipation that causes bedwetting to begin with.

Three Other Remedies to Avoid

The Internet offers no shortage of kooky bedwetting cures, and I won't address every ineffective treatment under the sun. Here are three popular remedies that won't help and can do harm.

Rewards Overactive bladders do not respond to the promise of M&Ms or extra screen time! Praise and rewards send the message that staying dry is within the child's control — which it's not — so kids are set up to feel like failures when they have an accident. (And this should go without saying, but children should never, ever be punished or shamed for having accidents.)

Limiting liquids Restricting fluids irritates the bladder and contributes to constipation, the very condition we're aiming to prevent. I'm not suggesting these kids guzzle Gatorade before bed, but they should drink plenty of water throughout the day.

Holding urine to "strengthen" the bladder Holding pee only exacerbates bedwetting, thickening and further irritating the bladder.

Do Bedwetting Alarms Work?

An alarm can train a child to wake up before wetting the bed, and this can be helpful. But it won't resolve the underlying constipation, so I recommend alarms only in addition to M.O.P., not as an alternative.

If you try the alarm, be patient! It can take up to three months for the child to reliably wake before wetting. Before then, a parent has to wake the child, help him change, and put the alarm back on. Some parents give up earlier out of exhaustion.

2 Lundmark E et al. Reboxetine in therapy-resistant enuresis: A randomized placebo-controlled study. J Pediatr Urol. 2016 Jul 12. pii: S1477-5131(16)30144-9.

PART 2

THE SCIENCE BEHIND M.O.P.

Clinical Nephrology, Vol. 23, No. 3 – 1985 (pp. 152–154)

Constipation, bladder instability, urinary tract infection syndrome

S. O'Regan, S. Yazbeck and E. Schick

Department of Pediatrics, Université de Montréal, Centre de Recherche Pediatrique, 3175, Chemin Côte Sainte-Catherine, Montreal, Québec, Canada H3T 1C5

Abstract. Forty-seven children with recurrent urinary tract infection were noted to have large fecal reservoirs by rectal examination and rectal manometry. Constipation was accompanied in the majority by enuresis and/or encopresis. Urodynamic studies indicated uninhibited bladder contractions. Aggressive treatment of the constipation resulted in cessation of infection in 44 patients, enuresis in 22 of 32 patients and encopresis in 20 of 21 patients and an improvement in bladder function with cessation of all other forms of treatment.

Key words: urinary tract infection – constipation – bladder contractions

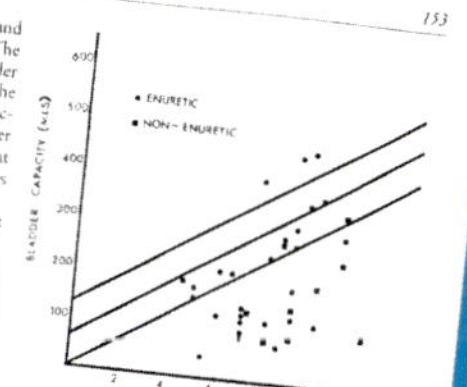

PART 2:

THE SCIENCE BEHIND M.O.P.

Science shows medication and bedwetting alarms are, at best, weak and unreliable methods of treating bedwetting.

And yet the medical establishment considers these the "first-line" treatments. On the other hand, science shows daily enemas to be highly effective — and yet this treatment is considered "too aggressive" or is not considered at all.

This makes no sense!

Doctors who object to daily enemas tend to fall into two groups: **1.)** those who don't believe constipation causes accidents (so what good would enemas do?), and **2.)** those who perceive enemas as too extreme, favoring oral laxatives instead.

Let's tackle both objections.

Proof Constipation is the Culprit

Dr. O'Regan was not the first to discover constipation causes bedwetting, but he was the first to prove it. I tell his fascinating story in *It's No Accident*. Here's the short version.

Back in the 1980s, Dr. O'Regan, a young father of three boys, was on a mission to figure out why his 5-year-old was wetting the bed. At the time, children who wet the bed were assumed to have either psychological or anatomic problems. Dr. O'Regan was sure his son had neither and turned to the McGill University Medical School library for answers. There he found research, dating back as far as the 1890s, that linked severe constipation with urinary problems.

Intrigued, Dr. O'Regan asked a colleague to assess whether his son was constipated, using a test called anal manometry. This is not a super fun test! A small balloon is inserted into the child's bottom and gradually inflated. The more inflation the child can tolerate, the more the rectum has been stretched by stool buildup. A child with normal rectal tone would notice the balloon inflated with just 5 to 10 ml of air, whereas a severely constipated child might not even detect the balloon until it's inflated with 40 ml of air.

"Seeing the X-ray really decreased our frustration with our son. We thought his accidents were a behavior or anxiety issue, but now we all have better attitudes, as we view the wetting as a medical issue."
– Mom of a 5-year-old

The O'Regan boy's results were astounding. Even when the balloon was fully inflated, to 110 ml, the size of a small tangerine, Dr. O'Regan's son felt no discomfort. As Dr. O'Regan's colleague noted, "The boy has no rectal tone."

Dr. O'Regan put his son on a regimen he predicted would clean out his rectum and restore its tone: enemas every night for a month, every other night for a second month, and twice a week for a third month. It worked. Within a week, the boy had his first dry night. Within two months, the bedwetting had stopped.

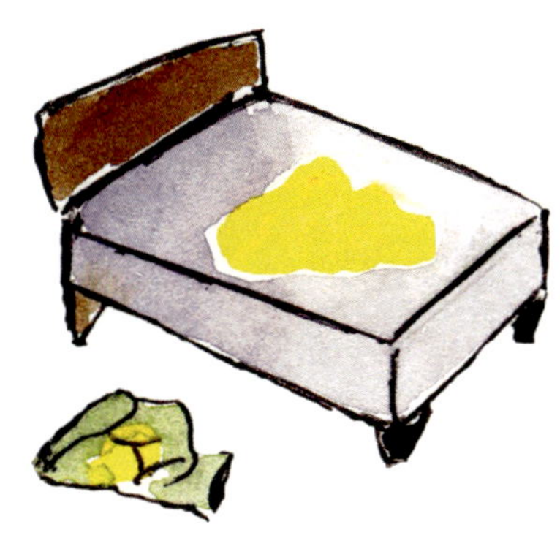

Contrary to popular belief, the cause of bedwetting is no mystery.

Buoyed by his success Dr. O'Regan began testing the regimen on hundreds of local children. The results of his studies (posted in full at BedwettingAndAccidents.com) were dramatic.

For example, in a study of 22 boys and girls with daytime and/or nighttime pee accidents, anal manometry showed all of them to be severely constipated. Seventeen of the families agreed to the enema regimen. The children achieved dryness within six weeks, on average. Nine months later, all but three were still accident free; those three had gone from having daily accidents to wetting once a week.[1]

In another study, this one tracking 47 girls with recurrent urinary tract infections, anal manometry showed the patients to be so constipated that every child could withstand 80 to 110 milliliters of air without discomfort. After the three-month enema regimen, 44 had stopped having UTIs. Of the subjects who also had encopresis, 20 of the 21 stopped pooping in their pants.[2] Of the girls with daytime wetting, 22 of the 32 stopped wetting. What about the girls who didn't improve? Most of their parents indicated they had not completed the enema regimen.

Dr. O'Regan was pleased to have discovered the cause of, and cure for, bedwetting, accidents, and recurrent UTIs. "These kids were told they were psychologically disturbed," he told me years later. "When you find something new that actually works, that makes a difference, it's quite spectacular."

And yet today, bedwetting is often considered a big mystery or a psychological issue. The National Institutes of Health states on its website[3]: "In most cases, the exact cause of bedwetting is not known." The NIH goes on to list "possible causes," including deep sleep, stress, an underdeveloped bladder, or urine overproduction.

Dr. O'Regan's studies made me curious about my own patients, so I began X-raying them as a matter of routine. (An X-ray is much easier, for both doctor and patient, than anal manometry!) What I've found: Well over 90% of my enuresis patients and 100% of my encopresis patients are severely constipated, defined as having a rectal diameter greater than 3 cm. Among children who do not have anatomic or neurologic problems (such as spina bifida) or type 1 diabetes (rare), it is clear that chronic constipation is virtually the only cause of wetting.

In one of my studies, published in Global Pediatric Health, we tracked 60 children with daytime wetting and found all were constipated. Their average rectal diameter was 6 cm, more than twice as wide as a healthy rectum.[4]

1 O'Regan S, Yazbeck S, Hamberger B, Schick E. Constipation a commonly unrecognized cause of enuresis. Am J Dis Child. 1986 Mar;140(3):260-1.
2 O'Regan S, Yazbeck S, Schick E. Constipation, bladder instability, urinary tract infection syndrome. Clin Nephrol. 1985 Mar;23(3):152-4.
3 https://www.niddk.nih.gov/health-information/health-topics/urologic-disease/urinary-incontinence-in-children/Pages/ez.aspx
4 Hodges SJ, Colaco M. Daily enema regimen is superior to traditional therapies for nonneurogenic pediatric overactive bladder. global pediatric health. 2016 (3) 1-4

3 Ways M.O.P. is "Modified"

Dr. O'Regan had remarkable success with his 90-day, step-down regimen. For years I had somewhat less success, probably because childhood constipation is more severe and more prevalent today than it was in Dr. O'Regan's time.

Childhood obesity rates have tripled since the 1980s, largely due to our kids' highly processed diet and low activity levels, two factors also driving the constipation epidemic. In addition, public school bathrooms today are scarier and filthier than they were in the 1980s, and school restroom policies are more restrictive, so fewer school-age kids are using the toilet at school.

Given all that, it does not surprise me that bedwetting and accidents are more difficult to resolve. In response to these trends, I have modified Dr. O'Regan's protocol in three ways, to keep the rectum clear longer and to make pooping easier. In my experience, these modifications boost the odds of success on M.O.P.

1) I recommend daily enemas for at least 30 days, tapering only after the child remains dry for at least 5 consecutive days.

Some children need daily enemas for more than 30 days before tapering.

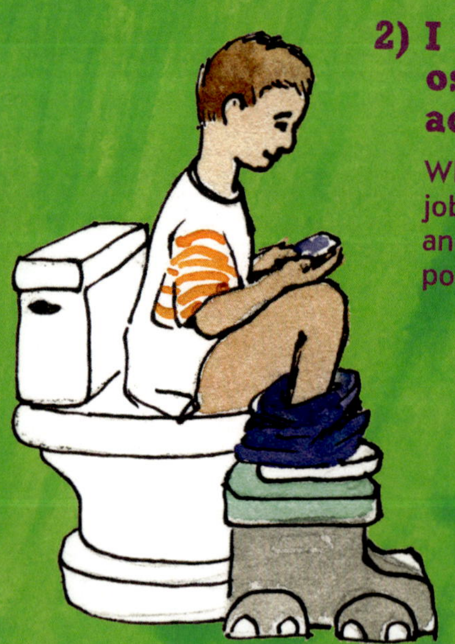

2) I recommend a daily osmotic laxative in addition to enemas.

Whereas enemas do a powerful clean-out job, osmotic laxatives such as MiraLAX and lactulose keep stool mushy, so pooping is less painful.

3) I recommend pooping with feet planted on a tall stool, to mimic the squatting position.

Squatting straightens the rectum, so poop empties more easily.

6 Mythical Causes of Bedwetting and Accidents

Here's a rundown of the most common explanations for bedwetting, all unproven or disproven.

> "Several doctors told us my daughter's accidents were due to behavior problems – hers and ours. One said, 'She could potty train if she wanted to. You need to figure out why she doesn't.' Another said, 'You need to be less involved in her bathroom routines – you've turned this into a power struggle. Parents shouldn't know how much their children are peeing and pooping.' "
>
> – Mom of 8-year-old

1) Deep sleep: Some studies show children who wet the bed are harder to wake than children who don't; others show they're not. But it doesn't matter, because deep sleep cannot explain why a child's bladder would be overactive at 3 a.m. Children with healthy bladders simply should not need to empty overnight.

So why don't these kids wake up before they pee? For the same reason, I believe, that children have daytime accidents: an overactive bladder spasms too quickly for the child to react. Even when fully awake, many kids can't make it to the toilet in time. So if a child is sleeping when the bladder hiccups, what chance does the child have of jolting awake and sprinting to the toilet in time to prevent an accident? None!

2) An underdeveloped bladder: Many parents are told their child's "bladder hasn't caught up with his brain." But there's no evidence that children who wet the bed have smaller bladders than other kids. Research does show these kids' bladders are more overactive. If the bladder of child who wets the bed has a smaller capacity to hold urine, that's because it's being squished by the stretched rectum.

3) Hormonal imbalance: Do some kids wet the bed because they overproduce urine overnight? Several studies have considered this theory, and none support it. That's why it makes no sense to treat bedwetting with drugs that trick the kidneys into producing less urine. Yet doctors prescribe these drugs all the time.

4) Stress or anxiety: Schools and doctors often refer these kids for therapy, and therapists often describe accidents as a reaction to "heartache" or "a lack of better communication tools." But it's usually accidents that cause stress, not the other way around. These kids get teased and shamed for a condition they can't control — they have plenty to feel stressed about. When I X-ray "stressed" kids, they're invariably constipated .

5) Laziness or attention seeking: There is zero evidence children have accidents because they can't be bothered to walk to the toilet. And given the amount of shame and blame heaped on these kids, you can be certain they are not seeking attention. If they are acting out, it's likely because they lack control over their bladder and/or bowels, and that feels crummy.

6) Heredity: It's true that kids with parents who wet the bed are more likely to wet the bed themselves. But that doesn't mean bedwetting is hereditary. More likely, the propensity toward constipation is passed down. I say this because when you X-ray kids who wet the bed, they're all stuffed with poop — not just the ones whose parents have a history of bedwetting.

Why Enemas Beat MiraLAX

Even if you're convinced constipation is causing your child's accidents, you may wonder: Do I really need to stick a tube up my child's bottom? Won't oral laxatives suffice?

In 2011, when *It's No Accident* was published, I was still advocating MiraLAX as an alternative to enemas for bedwetting and accidents. The book includes instructions for a high-dose MiraLAX clean-out, followed by a maintenance dose. *It's No Accident* does favor enemas, but since they are so unpopular and I'd seen OK results with MiraLAX, I felt it was a reasonable alternative.

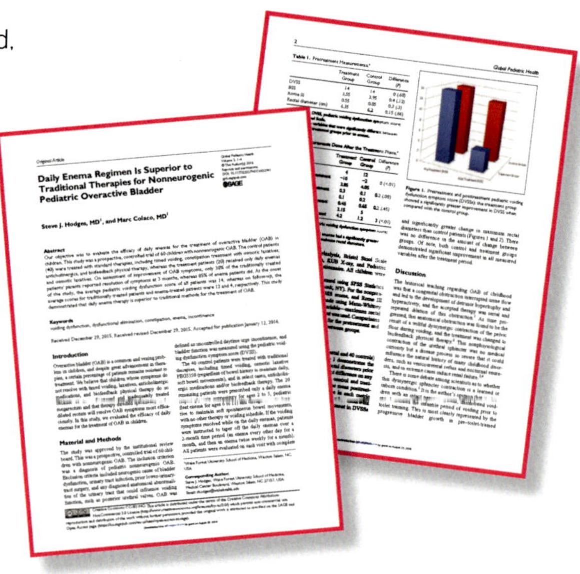

Original Article

Global Pediatric Health
Volume 3: 1–4
© The Author(s) 2016
SAGE

Daily Enema Regimen Is Superior to Traditional Therapies for Nonneurogenic Pediatric Overactive Bladder

Steve J. Hodges, MD[1], and Marc Colaco, MD[1]

Abstract

Our objective was to evaluate the efficacy of daily enemas for the treatment of overactive bladder (OAB) in children. This study was a prospective, controlled trial of 60 children with nonneurogenic OAB. The control patients (40) were treated with standard therapies, including timed voiding, constipation treatment with osmotic laxatives, anticholinergics, and biofeedback physical therapy, whereas the treatment patients (20) received only daily enemas and osmotic laxatives. On assessment of improvement of OAB symptoms, only 30% of the traditionally treated patients' parents reported resolution of symptoms at 3 months, whereas 85% of enema patients did. At the onset of the study, the average pediatric voiding dysfunction score of all patients was 14, whereas on follow-up, the average scores for traditionally treated patients and enema-treated patients were 12 and 4, respectively. This study demonstrated that daily enema therapy is superior to traditional methods for the treatment of OAB.

Keywords

voiding dysfunction, dysfunctional elimination, constipation, enema, incontinence

Received December 29, 2015. Received revised December 29, 2015. Accepted for publication January 12, 2016.

Introduction

Overactive bladder (OAB) is a common and vexing problem in children, and despite great advancement in therapies, a certain percentage of patients remains resistant to treatment. We believe that children whose symptoms do not resolve with timed voiding, laxatives, anticholinergic medications, and biofeedback physical therapy do so [illegible] and inadequately treated megarectum and that therapy directed [illegible] dilated rectum will resolve OAB symptoms most efficaciously. In this study, we evaluated the efficacy of daily enemas for the treatment of OAB in children.

Material and Methods

The study was approved by the institutional review board. This was a prospective, controlled trial of 60 children with nonneurogenic OAB. The inclusion criterion was a diagnosis of pediatric nonneurogenic OAB. Exclusion criteria included neurogenic cause of bladder dysfunction, urinary tract infection, prior lower-urinary-tract surgery, and any diagnosed anatomical abnormality of the urinary tract that could influence voiding function, such as posterior urethral valves. OAB was defined as uncontrolled daytime urge incontinence, and bladder function was measured using the pediatric voiding dysfunction symptom score (DVSS).

The 40 control patients were treated with traditional therapies, including timed voiding, osmotic laxative PEG3350 (regardless of bowel history to maintain daily, soft bowel movements), and in select cases, anticholinergic medications and/or biofeedback therapy. The 20 remaining patients were prescribed only a daily enema [illegible] for ages 2 to 5, pediatric fleet enema for ages 6 to 11) [illegible] tive to maintain soft spontaneous bowel movements, with no other therapy or voiding schedule. If the voiding symptoms resolved while on the daily enemas, patients were instructed to taper off the daily enemas over a 2-month time period (an enema every other day for a month, and then an enema twice weekly for a month). All patients were evaluated on each visit with complete

[1]Wake Forest University School of Medicine, Winston Salem, NC, USA

Corresponding Author:
Steve J. Hodges, Wake Forest University School of Medicine, Medical Center Boulevard, Winston Salem, NC 27157, USA.

My research shows that enemas work far better than traditional methods of resolving accidents.

I have changed my mind.

M.O.P. works so much better that I no longer recommend the MiraLAX route. Yes, a high-dose clean-out followed by months of a maintenance dose does work for some children. But the odds of success are so much lower than with **M.O.P.** MiraLAX is fine for treating constipated children who don't have accidents, but to resolve bedwetting or accidents, **M.O.P.** is the way to go.

In my *Global Pediatric Health* study, we tracked 60 patients, ages 4 to 11, who typically wet their pants daily. Forty of these patients followed standard therapies, including daily MiraLAX, a pee schedule, and, in some cases, medication. Another 20 patients agreed to daily enemas for at least 30 days before tapering, plus daily MiraLAX.

The results: After three months, 30% of the patients treated with standard therapies reported they'd stopped wetting, compared with 85% of the enema patients.

A close look at the data explains why enemas worked better. As I mentioned earlier, the average rectal diameter in both groups was greater than 6 cm at the start of the study. Three months later, the rectums of the 40 patients treated with standard therapy remained stretched — to 5 cm on average.

But the rectums of the enema group had rebounded dramatically — to 2.15 cm, on average. That's a completely normal measurement. Enemas clearly do a better job of cleaning out the rectum and of keeping it clear so it can heal.

MiraLAX, by contrast, often fails to dislodge the large, hard mass of stool clogging the rectum. Poop softened by MiraLAX may just ooze around the mass, so the problem doesn't resolve.

What about the three children in our enema group who did not stop wetting their pants? Unlike their peers, these patients were still stuffed with poop, according to our follow-up X-rays. Pediatric enemas simply weren't powerful enough to clear them out. For kids like them, I recommend large-volume enemas, described in Part 6.

Back in Dr. O'Regan's day, enemas were the only treatment for constipation — MiraLAX wasn't approved by the FDA until 1999. Today, enemas have fallen out of favor, and MiraLAX, available over the counter, is the go-to laxative. I understand why. It's easy to hand a child a glass of water mixed with a tasteless, odorless powder. It's not easy, at least at first, to insert a tube up a child's bottom.

But what makes more sense: doing what's easy or doing what works? MiraLAX does play a role in resolving accidents, but it works best as a supplement to, not a substitute for, daily enemas.

Yes, M.O.P. is Safe

I realize "daily enemas" just sounds unsafe. And I've had many patients report their physicians told them as much. But that is not a science-based observation!

In reality, enemas are safe as long as you limit them to once daily and your child is otherwise healthy. Dr. O'Regan tracked hundreds of patients who followed his regimen and reported no problems. My own experience also has shown **M.O.P.** to be safe.

Nonetheless, I understand the safety concerns. Here, I address the two most common safety questions.

Q: Could my child become dependent on enemas to poop?

A: No. There is absolutely no basis for this concern. In a child who has accidents, the rectum has become so stretched that it has lost the ability to contract and fully expel poop. Daily enemas give the rectum a chance to regain the sensation and strength to empty fully and regularly. Once that happens, the child will no longer need enemas.

One of the goals for a child on any version of **M.O.P.** is to poop spontaneously once a day, in addition to pooping after each enema. If the child is only pooping after enemas, this is NOT a sign of dependence on enemas; it just means the child hasn't fully regained rectal tone and/or sensation. Once the rectum bounces back, your child will be able to poop without enemas.

Q: Can enemas cause an electrolyte imbalance?

A: This is a worry that many doctors pass on to patients, but it is not supported by research. The theory is that since phosphorous, an electrolyte essential for the body's cells and organs to function, is included in over-the-counter enema solution, excess phosphorous will get absorbed into the child's body.

In reality, a child with normal kidney function will simply pee out the extra phosphorous. Any increase will be negligible. Complications from enemas are so uncommon that a review of 39 studies conducted over 50 years found a total of only 15 cases of electrolyte imbalance in children ages 3 through 18. Over 50 years.

"Our pediatrician said enemas are 'dangerous' and 'too risky' and that kids become dependent on them. What did she have to offer? She said my daughter should wear cotton underpants under her pull-ups at night so that she'd feel the wetness more and wake up."
— Mom of 7-year-old who got dry on M.O.P.

In nearly every case, the child had kidney disease or another chronic disease, was severely dehydrated, received multiple enemas in one day, or retained the enema fluid — or a combination of those factors. Retaining enema fluid is extremely rare in healthy children; it almost always happens in children with chronic medical conditions. I have never had a patient develop an electrolyte imbalance from enemas.

After prescribing enemas for years, I think concern among parents boils down to this: It just doesn't seem "natural" to insert anything into a child's bottom. Fair enough, but here's what else isn't natural: hauling around so much poop that you wet the bed, have accidents, or keep having UTIs.

M.O.P. Safety Guidelines:

1) Never perform enemas on a child with kidney disease.
2) If your child has another chronic disease, consult your doctor before doing enemas.
3) Never give a child more than one enema a day.
4) Make sure your child empties after the enema.

If, somehow, your child does not poop,
DO NOT administer another enema, and call your doctor. A child that clogged may have a serious condition requiring medical attention. But in virtually all cases, if you just wait, it'll happen.

PART 3

DIAGNOSING CONSTIPATION

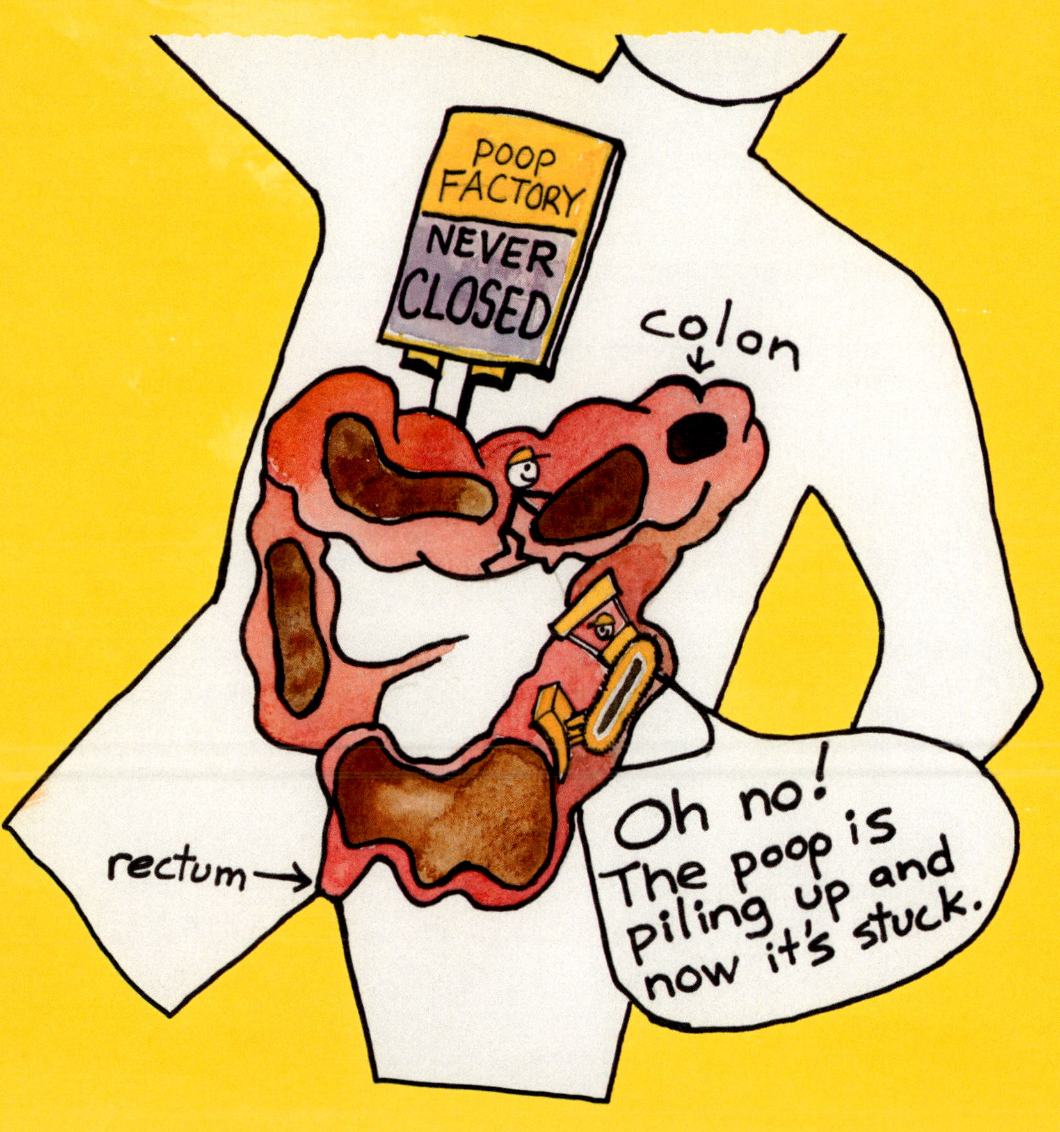

PART 3:
DIAGNOSING CONSTIPATION

Even doctors who know constipation causes wetting often fail to notice their patients are severely constipated.

I've had patients with grapefruit-sized rectal clogs that went unnoticed by the referring physician. I found these clogs because I X-ray all my enuresis patients. You simply can't argue with X-rays. They offer definitive proof that a child is (or isn't) constipated.

And yes, X-raying for constipation is safe.

Why Constipation Goes Unnoticed

Early in my career I diagnosed constipation using the methods I was taught in medical school: feeling the child's belly and asking how often the child poops. These methods are inadequate for two big reasons:

1.) **A severely constipated child may have a belly that looks and feels normal.** That's because the rectum just stretches to accommodate the extra poop. A small, wiry child can harbor massive amounts of poop without anyone noticing.

2.) **Many constipated children poop daily — they just don't fully evacuate.** So while infrequent pooping is a sign of constipation, the opposite isn't necessarily true: You can't assume a child who does poop daily is all clear.

This became obvious to me some years ago, when I would refer my toughest enuresis cases to gastroenterologists for evaluation. These GI docs would refer the patients right back to me, insisting these children were not constipated because they had normal "marker" studies. In other words, these patients would swallow capsules containing special markers that show up on an X-ray, and results would show these children's poop traveled through the colon in a timely manner. (This test is a fancier version of the popular "corn test" you can try at home: You eat corn, much of which is nondigestible, and track how long it takes for little yellow pieces to show up in your poop.)

Yet when I scrutinized the X-rays of the patients described by the GI doctor as "not constipated," I saw rectums full of poop. I realized what was happening: While some stool was passing through on a daily basis, it was oozing around the hard and growing lump that was aggravating the bladder.

"When I started X-raying my patients and could see how much their rectums were distended, I realized enemas were the only thing that would make a difference."
– James Sander, MD
Director of Pediatric Urology, Doctors Hospital at Renaissance, Edinburg, Texas

That's when I realized the conventional understanding of constipation is not relevant here. Constipation is typically defined as "having fewer than 3 bowel movements a week," but this is a faulty definition. It puts the emphasis on what is not happening (pooping) rather than what is happening: the rectum is being stretched by a giant mass of stool.

Dr. O'Regan recognized this definition problem and made note of it in his studies. He insisted on using anal manometry to detect constipation, knowing this procedure — invasive as it was — was the gold standard for detecting a stool pile-up and would tell the complete story. Urology textbooks from 40 years ago echo his recommendations. But somehow the message got lost, and today's guidelines simply recommend a patient exam and pooping history. No wonder constipation routinely flies under the radar.

X-raying for Constipation: A Game Changer

X-raying for constipation is not common medical practice, but for wetting patients, it should be. (There's no reason to X-ray for encopresis, since constipation is the only explanation.) We don't think twice about X-raying a child to diagnose a broken arm, an injury that will heal in six weeks. Yet many doctors won't X-ray to diagnose chronic constipation, a condition that can cause families years of suffering.

Some pediatricians maintain that X-rays pose an unwarranted health risk. One mom emailed me: "My son's pediatrician said an X-ray would expose my son to radiation that could later cause cancer." I strongly disagree. The radiation dose of an abdominal X-ray is the same dose you get from simply living for three months. The amount of good you can do for a child with bladder problems by accurately diagnosing constipation far outweighs the risks of a plain X-ray. Many parents don't grasp how a rectal clog can cause wetting until they see their child's flattened bladder on film.

If you absolutely don't want your child X-rayed but still want proof of constipation, you can have a pediatric GI clinic perform anal manometry, Dr. O'Regan's preferred method, or ultrasound. However, it's the rare ultrasound technician who has the skill and experience to scan for poop.

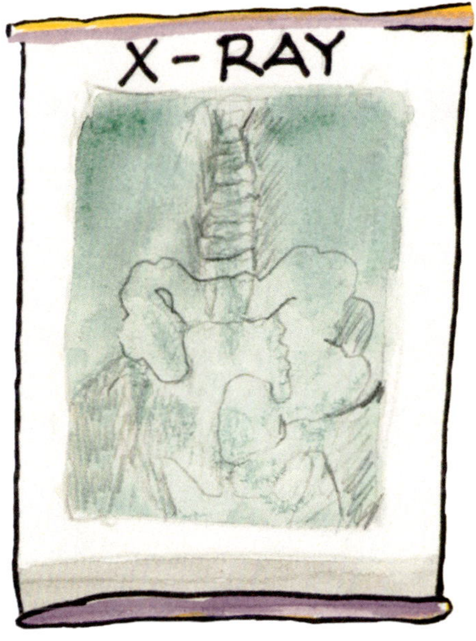

An X-ray offers proof that a child is (or isn't) constipated. Many parents are stunned to see how clogged their childs rectum is.

X-rays aren't necessary — many children on **M.O.P.** do not have access to them and do just fine. Still, X-rays can be valuable in numerous ways. Here are five.

1.) **X-rays confirm accidents aren't the child's fault.** When you look at an X-ray of a child's bladder being squished by a mass of poop, it just hits you: This kid has absolutely no control over the accidents. Many parents stop offering dryness rewards once they view their child's X-ray.

2.) **Children are more amenable to treatment.** Kids old enough to understand what an X-ray shows often become less resistant to enemas and to staying on a pee and poop schedule.

3.) **Skeptical doctors see the light.** Sometimes it's the doctor, not the parents, who needs convincing that a child is constipated and/or that more aggressive treatment is warranted. I've had countless parents tell me their pediatricians agreed to enemas after reviewing X-rays.

4.) **You have a baseline for later comparison.** I don't routinely order second X-rays, but when a child has been on **M.O.P.** for 30 days without progress, a follow-up X-ray can help guide the course of treatment. Usually, the child is still full of poop and requires more powerful enemas.

5.) **You know to search for another cause if constipation is ruled out.** Every once in a blue moon, an X-ray shows a patient's rectum to be normal. That's when I know to look for another cause, such as an anatomic blockage of the bladder or a neurological problem.

How to Read an X-ray for Constipation

I regularly read X-rays from parents seeking a second opinion. "The doctor didn't think there was any blockage," a mom will write. "What do you see?" More often than not, I see a very large and obvious mass of stool in the rectum.

Why do so many doctors miss the blockage? Because they don't know where to look. They may tell parents, "The colon will always contain some stool, so what we see here doesn't mean anything." But it does. While it's true that the colon will always contain some poop, the primary place to look for excess stool is the rectum. If it's greater than 3 cm in diameter, the child is constipated. Most of my wetting patients have rectums wider than 6 cm.

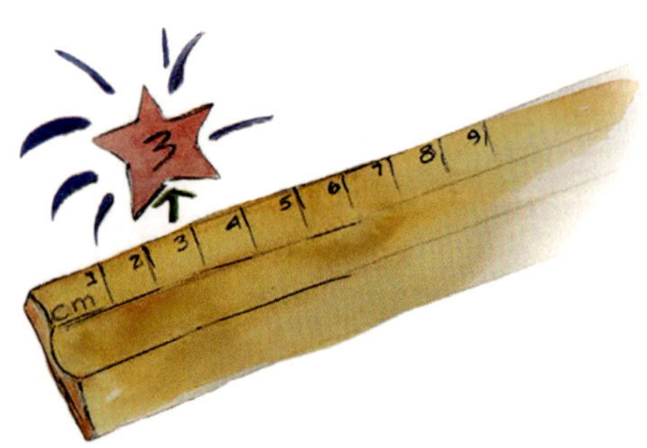

A rectal diameter exceeding 3 cm indicates constipation

Many wetting patients also have excess stool in the ascending colon, the section that pushes poop up against gravity. Make sure your doctor reads your child's X-ray, rather than relying on a report from a radiologist. Radiologists don't always comment on stool burden, so they may miss it. If your doctor insists your child's X-ray is normal, ask for a measurement of the rectal diameter.

Why Our Kids Are Clogged

Potty accidents are the last topic anyone wants to talk about at the park or on social media, but you can be assured your family has loads of company in your struggle with accidents. One-fourth of American 5-year-olds wet the bed or have daytime accidents, and each year, half a million kids visit the doctor for these issues. In recent years, hospital clinics have reported big increases in the number of children treated for constipation. Kindergarten teachers have expressed concern that more students are having accidents in class. This isn't just happening in the United States but also in Westernized countries around the world.

The potty-problem epidemic is global.

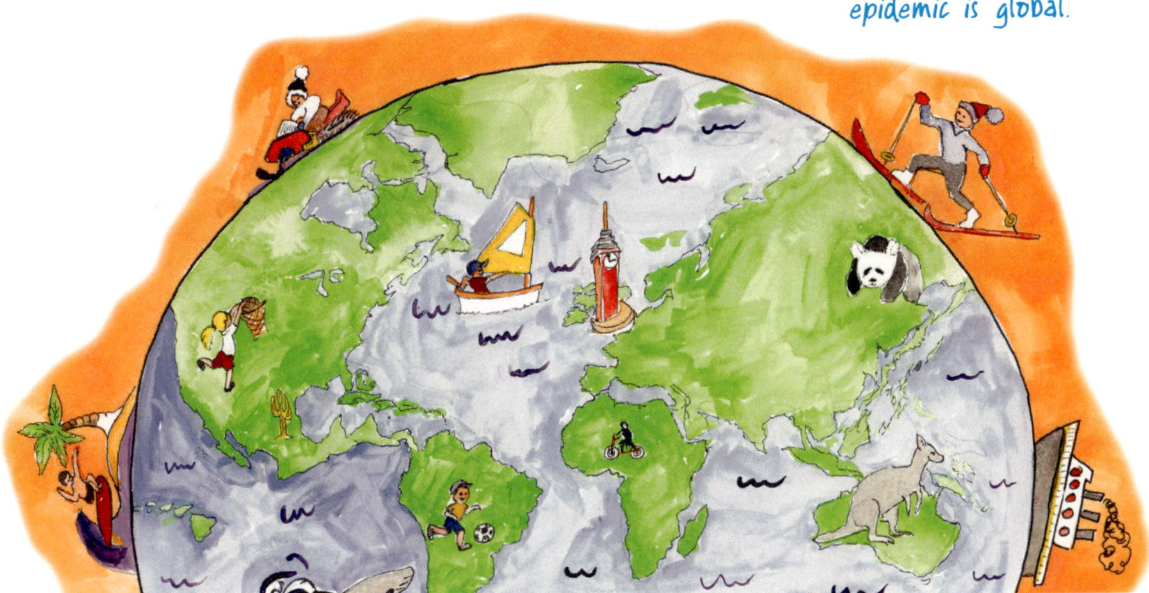

What the heck is going on?

Unbelievably, parental laziness is often blamed for the rise in accidents. In an article from a Manchester, England, newspaper, a potty training "expert" says, "No one is taking responsibility for potty training. Parents say they expect the nursery to do it, while the nursery thinks the parents will do it." In response to a Washington Post article about a child suspended from preschool for accidents, an online commenter called the mother "a lazy person who wants to dump the kid off [at preschool] so she can shop and drink Starbucks." Another commenter said the mother should "quit blaming others for her failures."

Blaming parents is ludicrous and demonstrates zero understanding of the societal forces contributing to our epidemic of childhood constipation. In *It's No Accident* I explain these forces in detail. Here I will summarize the four main causes of widespread constipation.

1.) The highly processed Western diet: Babies on breast milk or formula have mushy poop. Life is good! It's only when they start on solid foods — especially the highly processed products marketed to children — that their stool becomes hard and painful to pass. So even before toilet training, many children have developed the habit of withholding.

In her book *100 Days of Real Food*, Lisa Leake recalls that one of her daughters completely overcame constipation when the family cut out processed food. Not surprising! If eating "real food" were the norm in Westernized countries, no doubt rates of constipation, bedwetting, and accidents would be dramatically lower. But as a culture, we have a long way to go. (Read Michael Moss's book *Salt Sugar Fat: How the Food Giants Hooked Us* to get an idea of just how far we are from that ideal.)

I am often asked: Could dietary intolerances contribute to constipation? Sure, that may be the case with some children. If you suspect an intolerance to milk or wheat or anything else, it's worth experimenting with your child's diet to see if that makes a difference. Just recognize that if a child is already having accidents, dietary changes won't suffice; it will take enemas to resolve the hardened mass of stool stretching the rectum.

2.) The rush to potty train: As a father of three, I know what a happy day it is when a child graduates from diapers. Sayonara, stinky diaper bag! And I understand that it's convenient for preschools to have classes full of potty-trained 3-year-olds. But our culture is in too big a hurry to toilet train, and this rush leads to countless cases of constipation.

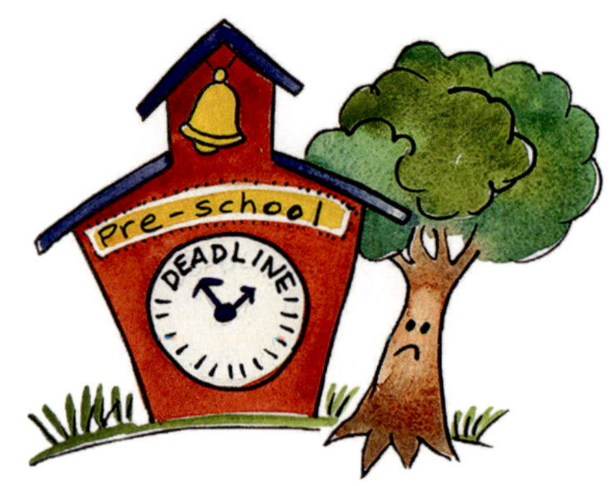

Preschool potty-training deadlines prompt many parents to train their children before they are ready, increasing the risk these kids will develop wetting problems.

As my published research shows, children trained before age 2 have triple the risk of developing wetting problems than children trained later.[1] Based on my clinical experience, I do not advise training until around age 3. Yet many preschools won't accept 3-year-olds in pull-ups, forcing many parents to train their children as toddlers.

Problem is, 2-year-olds don't understand how important it is to use the toilet when nature calls. They think you dash to the bathroom only when you desperately need to! At preschool these newly trained kids often feel too shy to tell the teacher they need to use the toilet. Or, they're too excited by all the fun or worried that another kid will abscond with their toy truck while they're in the bathroom. So instead of heeding the urge to pee or poop, they ignore it time and again, eventually becoming expert holders.

The consequences may not become apparent for two or three years down the line, when their constipation becomes severe enough to trigger accidents.

Among my missions is to persuade preschools to relax their toilet-training mandates. I frequently write letters on behalf of students who have been threatened with suspension for accidents, and I see firsthand how these mandates can backfire, causing families much distress.

A typical preschool policy reads: "If a child has multiple accidents in a day or over a period of days, and we realize a child is not fully toilet trained, then we may ask that parents keep the child home for a week or two to complete toilet learning." If accidents persist, these policies state, families may be asked to leave school.

Policies like these may sound reasonable, but they are based on a fundamental misunderstanding of toileting accidents. Sending these kids home for a week to "work on" their potty skills is like sending dyslexic children home for a week to work on their reading. It's going to fail, because accidents have nothing to do with lack of training.

1 Hodges SJ, Richards KA, Gorbachinsky I, Krane LS. The association of age of toilet training and dysfunctional voiding. *Research and Reports in Urology*. 2014 Oct. (6): 127-130

When you let children lead the way on toilet training rather than dictate what month they will be trained, their risk of developing peeing and pooping problems diminishes greatly.

3.) Minimal potty-training follow-up: Once children are toilet trained, we tend to stop paying attention to their peeing and pooping habits. But potty training is the time when parents (and preschool teachers) must pay the most attention, because once the holding habit takes root, it's difficult to reverse.

Potty training isn't a skill, like riding a bike, that gets locked in once things "click." Learning to poop on the toilet is different from learning to heed your body's urge to poop. The latter requires daily reinforcement, and that's not part of our culture.

Sure, we pay cursory attention: When we see kids doing the "potty dance," crossing their legs and curtsying, we insist they go pee. When we notice they haven't pooped in a while, we tell them to try. But we don't explain *why*.

Preschoolers are capable of understanding what healthy poop looks like and what happens to the bladder and colon when you hold your pee and poop. If healthy toileting were taught in preschool and reinforced in grade school, and if we monitored our kids for the subtle signs of constipation, we would have a lot fewer cases of encopresis and enuresis.

4.) Restrictive school bathroom policies: Even kids who survive preschool without becoming constipated can develop wetting problems once they hit the school system. I have huge numbers of patients who go from 7:30 a.m. to 3:30 p.m. without using the toilet.

Some of these kids are too grossed out, scared, or embarrassed to use school bathrooms. They report stalls littered with toilet paper, walls marred by graffiti, sinks with no paper towels or soap, toilet water that's yellow or brown.

But more commonly, children run up against classroom policies that encourage holding. Some 36% of elementary teachers reward students who don't use bathroom passes or punish those who do, according to a University of California at San Francisco survey of more than 4,000 teachers. Fully 76% of teachers implement policies that undermine their students' toileting health. This is not surprising, as only 18% of teachers receive training in healthy toileting practices for children.

At some schools, students earn restroom passes for good behavior. Other schools dangle prizes for not using bathroom passes. Students can earn trinkets, "money" for the student store, even pizza parties — all for ignoring their bodies' signals.

Many schools lock restrooms at lunchtime or after school, when kids head to the bus (never mind that students may have a 45-minute ride home), and they close bathrooms in response to behavior problems.

Many students are too grossed out, scared, or embarrassed to use school bathrooms, so they hold from 7:30 a.m. to 3:30 p.m.

Interestingly, the UCSF teachers survey was coauthored by a physician, Lauren Ko, who formerly taught second grade at a Bronx school that limited bathroom access. She told me: "I noticed kids having accidents in the classroom, and I know it was really humiliating for them."

> "Using the bathroom is a biological necessity, not a privilege to be earned or denied."
> – Mom of middle-schoolers who earned bathroom passes for good behavior

In defending their policies, many schools and teachers insist that students typically ask to use the bathroom for reasons unrelated to biology — as one former teacher put it to me, "boredom, curiosity, to play around in the bathroom, because their friend needed to go, to get out of doing other things."

Posting on Facebook, she continued: "I don't get up during meetings to go to the restroom. That's not how life works, people." Yikes, harsh! This person is an adult—with a fully grown bladder, unlimited bathroom access, and no fear of being bullied in a restroom stall at lunchtime.

I know teachers have the very tough job of managing a classroom on top of countless other stresses, and no doubt some students will try to game the system. But if students who claim they have to pee are in fact roaming the hallways up to no good, surely measures can be taken that are unrelated to restricting bodily functions.

Students must be allowed to use the restroom when the urge arises—not 10 or 20 or 60 minutes later. It's a health issue, and it's no joke.

A Culture That Promotes Toileting Problems

Why did your child become constipated to the point of having accidents? Probably some combination of the factors I just listed, although some kids are just unlucky. I've known many kids who, because of their genetics or temperaments, manage to avoid toileting problems, despite eating tons of processed foods, toilet training as toddlers, and steering clear of school bathrooms. I also have patients who love broccoli and potty trained at age 3 and still developed problems.

But the fact remains: Enough forces in our culture conspire against healthy toileting behaviors that an astonishing numbers of kids end up with whacked-out bladders.

PART 4

STARTING M.O.P.

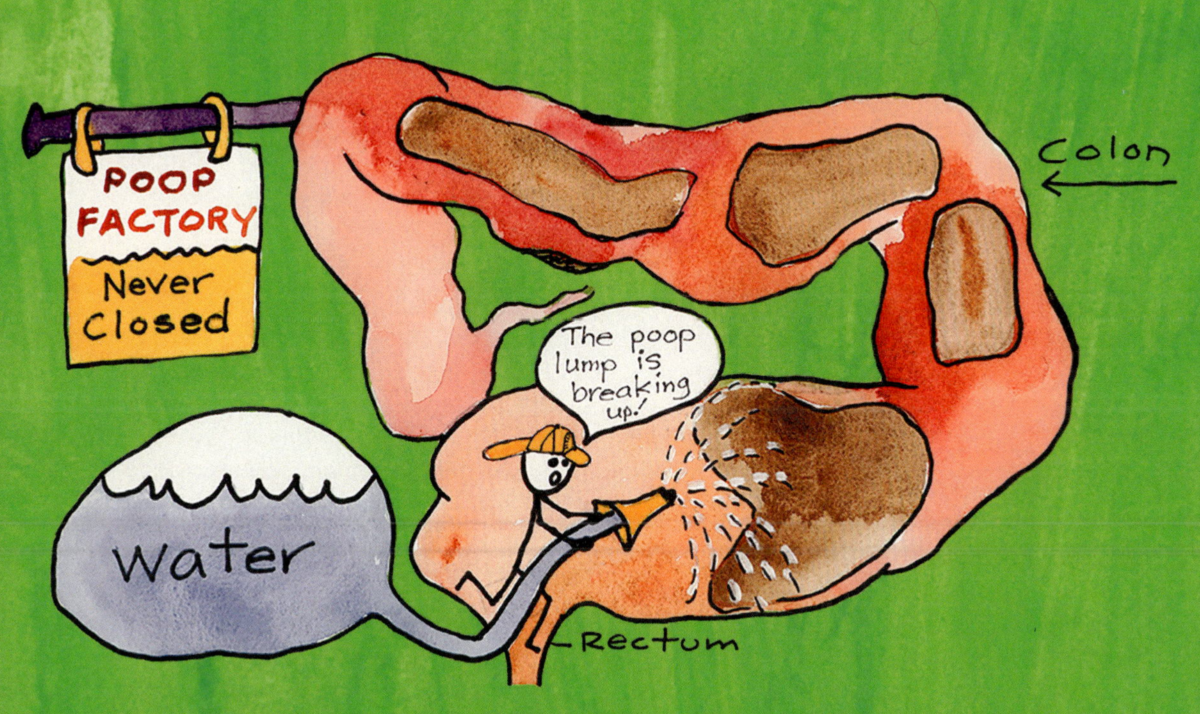

PART 4:

STARTING M.O.P.

It's always helpful to work with a healthcare provider when your child is on M.O.P.

Every child's case is unique, and a doctor or nurse practitioner may have insight into your child's circumstances that could influence how you approach enemas.

Also, with a doctor on board, you can get baseline and (if necessary) follow-up X-rays, as well as prescriptions for lactulose (an alternative to MiraLAX) and any other medications you may need.

However, many doctors don't know how well enemas work, don't believe they are helpful, or are downright hostile to them. If your doctor won't budge, I recommend finding a more informed healthcare provider or going ahead on your own. Enemas don't require a prescription or expertise to administer, and countless families have successfully completed **M.O.P.** without a problem.

In this part, I offer ideas on gaining your doctor's buy-in, discuss supplies needed, and get into the nitty-gritty of giving a child an enema.

Getting Your Doctor on Board

Many parents have told me that completing M.O.P. was a breeze compared to getting their doctor's approval. One mom emailed that her pediatrician said, "Enemas will emotionally scar your daughter for life." Another mom posted on our Facebook page, "When I brought enemas up to our doctor, he said, 'There's no way I would do that to my child.'"

Yet another mom posted that when she reported positive **M.O.P.** results to her pediatrician, "She said I had to 'stop that right away.'" The doctor's recommendation? That the parents offer their daughter rewards for dry nights and that the child wear cotton underwear underneath her pullups so she would "feel the wetness more and wake up."

This mom asked me: "How is a mom supposed to stand up to a pediatrician who doesn't know anything about this?"

Good question!

Sometimes you just can't. Some doctors — not just pediatricians but my fellow pediatric urologists, too — simply will never get on board. I know this from experience, as I myself often have difficulty persuading my colleagues that constipation causes bedwetting and that enemas are superior to MiraLAX.

With some physicians, no amount of scientific research, case studies, or good reports from parents will change their minds. As one mom posted, when she reported her daughter had gone from five accidents per day to one or zero while on **M.O.P.**, the pediatrician said it was "just coincidence" and the girl was "growing out of it."

But other doctors have proven to be more open-minded. Here are a few ideas for gaining a skeptical doctor's support for X-rays and/or M.O.P..

- **Explain the toll that accidents are taking on your family.** Doctors who suggest waiting it out or using MiraLAX may not realize how stressful and frustrating your child's accidents are for everyone. Try: "This is difficult for our family. We are brainstorming different possibilities. In our research, we came across this. . . "
- **Bring published research**. Doctors may not be interested in reading our books or blog posts, but they might be willing to glance at published scientific research. If your doctor pushes MiraLAX, download "Daily Enema Regimen Is Superior to Traditional Therapies for Nonneurogenic Pediatric Overactive Bladder," from the Research page of my website. If your doctor disagrees that constipation causes bedwetting, download Dr. O'Regan's studies from my website, as well as the Journal of Urology comment by Angelique Champeau, RN, director of the Children's Continence Clinic at UCSF Benioff Children's Hospital. In the comment she writes: "After 16 years of managing urinary tract dysfunction in children, I would hypothesize that the number [of cases caused by constipation] is closer to 90-100%. Using a prevalence of 50% can cause gross under-treatment."

  You might also note that our books are endorsed by the pediatric urology departments at both UCSF and the Mayo Clinic.
- **Ask for research.** Flip things around: If your doctor pushes more MiraLAX or maintains enemas are traumatizing, mention that you'd like to read up on that. Ask the doctor to point you to some studies on the subject.
- **Ask lots of questions.** For example: "Have enemas been traumatizing for other patients?" "Do you have any experience with M.O.P. or a similar regimen?"
- **Take the "humor me" approach**. If your doctor assures you your child is not constipated, insist on an X-ray and indicate you'll try a different approach if your child's rectal diameter proves to be under 3 cm.

M.O.P. Supply List

Here are tips for choosing and purchasing the supplies needed for M.O.P.: enemas, an osmotic laxative, and a tall toilet stool.

Enemas

Best-case scenario, you will need 53 enemas: 30 for the first month, 15 for the second month, and 8 for the third month. However, if your child is not totally dry by day 30, you will need to continue with daily enemas until dryness. So, you may end up needing more than 53 enemas.

Yikes, that's a lot! I recommend buying them in bulk online. Your pharmacy may even resist selling you the number you need for M.O.P.. Some doctors we work with receive phone calls from stunned pharmacists asking, "Are you sure you prescribed 30 enemas?"

Any brand is fine, but you may want to experiment. Some children find the tips of certain brands more comfortable than those of other brands. Adding petroleum jelly to the tip and to the child's bottom should alleviate discomfort. Some kids feel a burning sensation from the phosphorous solution found in pediatric enemas and prefer the pure saline or glycerin enemas used in our M.O.P.+ program (described in Part 6). Or, you can switch to liquid glycerin suppositories, pediatric size for children age 6 and under and adult size for children age 6 and older.

Osmotic laxatives

Osmotic laxatives - such as MiraLAX, lactulose, or Pedia-Lax chewable tablets - serve a different purpose from enemas. Whereas enemas flush out the clog and keep the rectum clear on a daily basis, osmotic laxatives draw water into the colon to keep stool mushy, so pooping is less painful. Children on **M.O.P.** should poop daily on their own, not just right after the enema, and the poop should come out like soft-serve ice cream. That's where laxatives help.

> "Our pediatrician and pediatric gastroenterologist considered M.O.P. excessively aggressive, but after reading Dr. Hodges' research, I determined that enemas sounded less messy and made more sense than doing the MiraLAX cleanout. We moved forward on our own, with great success."
> – Mom of a 5-year-old

Osmotic laxatives differ from stimulant laxatives, such as Ex-Lax. These laxatives, which may be helpful for some children, stimulate the intestinal muscles to contract and squeeze out the idle poop. They should be prescribed by a physician, as they can be habit-forming in high doses over extended periods.

Osmotic laxatives, on the other hand, are not habit-forming and are safe for extended periods of time — months, even years, if necessary.

Below I describe three reliable osmotic laxatives for kids: PEG 3350 powder (MiraLAX), lactulose, and chewable laxative tables with magnesium hydroxide. Many parents swear by other laxatives, such as magnesium citrate liquid, and if you find one that works for your child, I say: Go for it! I don't have strong feelings about which osmotic laxative to use. What matters is keeping poop mushy. Your child can take the full dose once a day or take half a dose twice a day.

MiraLAX or generic equivalent: Key ingredient: PEG 3350, polyethylene glycol, a synthetic compound

Pros: A flavorless, odorless powder sold in large bottles, MiraLAX is easy to administer. You simply mix it in water or other clear liquids.

Cons: Some kids may resist drinking as much liquid as they need to, and for a minority of kids, PEG 3350 just doesn't work well. More significantly, questions have been raised over MiraLAX safety.

More than 100 studies have found PEG 3350 is safe for children, even babies, and none have linked MiraLAX to severe or harmful side effects. Virtually every pediatrician in America routinely prescribes MiraLAX. However, scientists are investigating whether PEG 3350 may cause psychiatric problems in children, as the U.S. Food and Drug Administration has occasionally received reports of tremors and obsessive-compulsive behavior in children given PEG 3350.

What do I think? I welcome all research but am inclined to think MiraLAX is safe for the relatively short duration of **M.O.P.** In my experience, the side effects — flatulence, nausea, abdominal cramping — are rare and minor. The MiraLAX bottle indicates that vomiting is also a possible side effect, although it's not something parents have reported to me.

Lactulose: Key ingredient: Lactose, a non-absorbable, manufactured sugar that contains two naturally occurring sugars, galactose and fructose

Pros: Some children respond better to this sweet, syrupy liquid than they do to MiraLAX. Also, some children are more willing to swallow two teaspoons of a sweet liquid than a glass full of liquid.

Cons: Lactulose requires a prescription. Its side effects — diarrhea, nausea, gas — are the same as those associated with MiraLAX.

Laxative chews (such as Pedia-Lax Chewable Tablets): Key ingredient: magnesium hydroxide, a saline laxative also known as milk of magnesia

Pros: For some kids, chewable tablets are more convenient than mixing laxative powder.

Cons: If your child requires a lot of laxative to maintain mushy poop, chews may get expensive. Also, some children don't like the taste. The most common side effect is diarrhea.

Toilet Stool

You probably haven't thought about a toilet stool since your child was potty training. But children of every age — and adults, too, for that matter! — should place their feet on a stool when pooping. The stool should be tall enough to place your child in a squatting position.

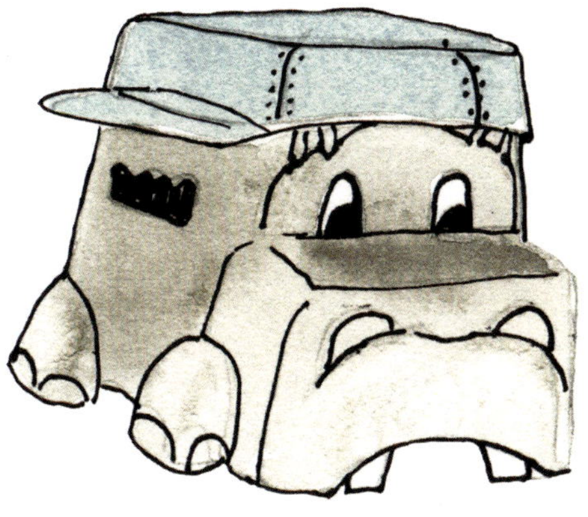

It's important for constipated children to poop with their feet firmly planted on a tall stool.

Fact is, human beings were designed to squat while pooping. Squatting straightens the rectum, letting poop fall out easily. If you've ever pooped in the woods, you know what I'm talking about! By contrast, sitting upright is like trying to poop uphill. With the rectum bent, poop has a tougher exit.

Studies even show that pooping in a squatting position is more comfortable and faster. In one study, subjects took 2 minutes and 10 seconds to poop while sitting on a tall toilet, compared to 51 seconds in a squatting position.[1] What's more, toilets are too tall for children. With their feet dangling, kids often clench their inner thighs and can't relax. Think about it: Do you fully relax your body when you're sitting on a barstool without a footrest? No!

In addition, make sure your child sits on a kid-sized toilet seat, either a flip-down seat or one that you place on the rim. When kids sit on an adult-sized toilet, they clench their pelvic-floor muscles to keep from falling in. We can't see them doing it, and they may not even know they are doing it, but I assure you, they are!

1 Sikirov, D. "Comparison of straining during defecation in three positions: results and Implications for human health." Digestive Diseases and Sciences.Vol. 48, No. 7, 1201-1205

M.O.P. Guidelines

Here, as a reminder, are the five M.O.P. guidelines. I recommend toilet-trained children age 3 and under use pediatric liquid glycerin suppositories instead of pediatric enemas. For children age 4+, pediatric enemas tend to work best, though some older kids respond better to liquid glycerin suppositories.

Children on **M.O.P.** should eventually poop once a day on their own, in addition to pooping after the enema.

1: Do daily enemas for at least 30 days.
- Taper only when the child remains dry for at least 5 consecutive days

2: After 30 days and 5 consecutive days of dryness, do enemas every other day for a month.
- If accidents recur, return to daily enemas.

3: After a second 30 days of dryness, do enemas twice a week for one month before stopping.
- If accidents recur, return to daily enemas.

4: Take a daily osmotic laxative to keep poop mushy. Continue the daily laxative throughout M.O.P. and for 3 to 6 months after.

5: Poop with feet on a stool.
- The stool must be tall enough to place the child in a squatting position.

Giving an Enema in 5 Easy Steps

You can administer the enema on a bed or, for less potential mess, on the floor near the toilet. Any time of day is fine, though for most families bedtime tends to be less disruptive to their schedule.

The following directions apply to store-bought pediatric enemas. For instructions on administering homemade enemas, see Part 6.

What you need: a pediatric enema (squeeze bottle, tube, lubricated tip) and petroleum jelly

Wash your hands before you remove the enema from the box, and then follow these steps.

"Our doctor said enemas would create trauma for my son, which has not been our experience at all. He enjoys his iPad time, and it's just part of our evening routine, like brushing teeth. My son feels so much better not being stuffed up that he doesn't mind them at all."
– Mom of 9-year-old

Step 1: **Show your child the bottle, tube, lubricated tip, and extra lubrication.** Explain what you're about to do, and briefly review why.

If your child worries the tube will hurt, explain that the extra lubrication will help the tube slide in more easily. You might also point out that anus is quite stretchy and the tip is smaller than any BM a constipated child has pooped out!

Step 2: **Place a towel on the floor or bed, and instruct the child to lie on the left side,** knees bent toward the chest. Because of the colon's anatomy, lying on the left side helps the emptying process.

Step 3: **Rub petroleum jelly on your child's anus and/or add lubrication to the tip.** Insert the tip straight in the child's bottom, making sure it gets past the sphincter.

You'll know you are in when you pass the point of resistance and when you squeeze and no liquid leaks back. Encourage your child to take deep breaths — like blowing out birthday candles or blowing up a balloon — to help relax the sphincter. Tensing up can make the process uncomfortable.

Step 4: **Squeeze the bottle slowly and steadily until you have squeezed as much as directed by your doctor or the package.**

Enema companies recommend using half a bottle for children 2 to 5 and a full bottle (or as directed by a doctor) for children 5 to 11. Enema bottles have a one-way valve, so you can release and squeeze again to make sure you've squeezed out all the liquid.

If your child's rectum is so stuffed with poop that the enema liquid stretches it to the point of pain, stop and encourage your child to poop. The discomfort should diminish with each day, as the rectum empties.

Step 5: **When nearly all the solution has been flushed into your child's rectum, remove the tube.** Bottles typically contain slightly more liquid than is needed.

Your child can either sit on the toilet right away or remain seated or lying until she feels the urge to poop, ideally in 5 to 10 minutes. (The child may have to work up to holding that long.) Even if your child poops enough for a whole soccer team, stick with the regimen. There's likely more where that came from!

Dosing Osmotic Laxatives

Have your child take an osmotic laxative at roughly the same time each day. Or divide the dose and have the child take half in the morning and half at night.

Finding the right dose can take trial and error. To achieve mushy poop, some kids need a lot more laxative than others. Evaluate your child's poop consistency yourself, when possible, as second-hand reports from 5-year-olds are often unreliable. Older children are more reliable — and probably won't want you inspecting their poop! — so have them report back using our "How's Your Poop?" chart on page 40.

Keep your child on the full laxative dose for 3 to 6 months after dryness. At that point, gradually cut the dose in half for two weeks. Then give your child half a dose every other day for two weeks, and then every third day for two weeks. Then stop. If at any time your child seems backed up again, go back one step.

MiraLAX or generic equivalent: Start with one capful (17 grams) a day, mixed in 4 to 8 ounces of a clear liquid, such as water, juice, or Gatorade. Taking half a capful twice a day is fine.

Mix until the drink is completely clear. You shouldn't see particles of powder floating around. If your child's poop is firmer than total mush, increase the dose by ¼ to ½ a capful per day. If your child is pooping diarrhea, decrease the dose by ¼ to ½ capful. Continue to monitor poop consistency and adjust as necessary.

Lactulose: I typically prescribe 10 grams of lactulose once a day (or 5 ml twice a day) for starters and advise parents to adjust as needed.

Chews: Experiment in the range of 3 to 6 tablets daily.

Pooping Tips

Instruct your child to lean forward while pooping. Also: elbows on knees, shoulders rounded but spine straight, and tailbone pushed out rather than tucked. I know it sounds like some complicated yoga pose, but it's pretty simple and can make a big difference. This position places the rectum in a vertical position, giving your child the benefit of gravity, and stretches the abdominal cavity, giving the colon more room to pump stool to the rectum for emptying.

All children should poop with their feet firmly planted on a toilet stool, and smaller kids should sit on a toilet seat. With no worries about falling in, children are better able to relax and fully empty.

PART 5

TRACKING YOUR CHILD ON M.O.P.

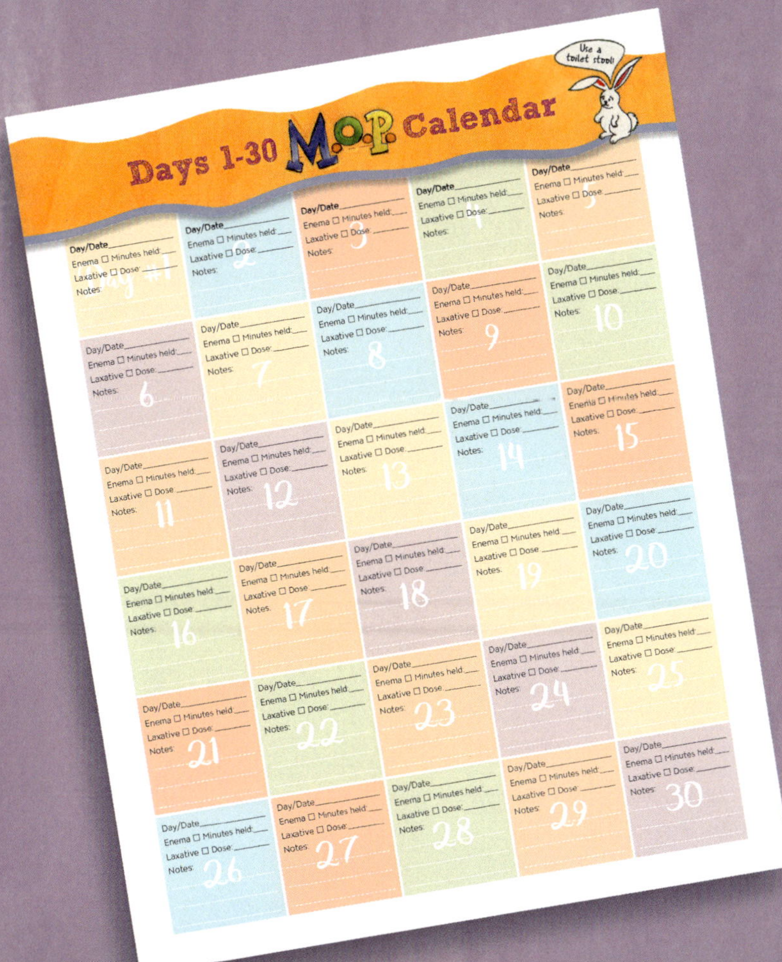

PART 5:

TRACKING YOUR CHILD ON M.O.P.

I know M.O.P. is a big undertaking, and I don't want to make it bigger by suggesting you take copious notes on your child's progress!

However, some basic tracking will alert you to patterns in your child's symptoms, and these patterns will help you make decisions about how to proceed.

It is important to re-evaluate your child's progress on **M.O.P.** every 30 days. I've received emails from parents who say, "I did **M.O.P.** for 6 months, and it didn't work." Whoa! If your child is making zero progress after 30 days, you need to make a change, like switching to large-volume enemas or adding glycerin to the enema solution. There's always a next step to try, so don't stick with an approach that isn't working.

On the other hand, don't dismiss small signs of improvement. Some signs, like less urgency to pee or more spontaneous pooping (other than after an enema) — are subtle and suggest you should stay the course even when wetting persists.

Of course, tracking dry nights will let you know when to start tapering from daily enemas. Some families, in their excitement to complete the protocol, taper too soon, paving the way for a relapse. Some kids relapse for no discernible reason, and you simply need to start over, discouraging as that prospect may be.

Keeping notes will also help your family remember to stick with the regimen each day. As one mom told me, "It seems like it would be easy to remember whether you gave your child an enema or when you switched to a new type of solution, but it's not!" An occasional missed day won't matter, but skipping enemas more often may compromise your results.

You can track your child's progress in a notebook, on your computer, or on our **M.O.P.** tracker — whatever works for you. Use the poop chart on page 40 to assess the consistency of your child's poop.

M.O.P. Tracking Tips

Here is some guidance on filling in each section of the tracking calendar.

Enema/minutes held: Check off the enema, and note how many minutes your child held in the solution before pooping. It can take practice for a child to hold enemas for the recommended 10 minutes. Children who can only hold for 2 or 3 minutes may not be getting the full benefit of the enema.

If your child has an easy time holding for 10 minutes and still doesn't feel the urge to poop, it's time to switch to large-volume enemas or add glycerin and/or castile soap to the large-volume saline solution. See Part 6 for details.

Laxative/dosage: Check off whether your child took a laxative, and note the dosage taken (for example: "1 cap MiraLAX"). Tracking the dosage can help you make adjustments until you hit that sweet spot: poop that's mushy but not runny.

Notes: Depending on your child's symptoms, note any of the following:

- **Number of accidents (bedwetting, daytime pee, and/or poop)**
- **Number of poops other than after enema**
- **Belly pain**
- **Ability to sense the urge to poop**
- **Pee frequency**
- **Pee urgency**
- **Presence/absence of skid marks**

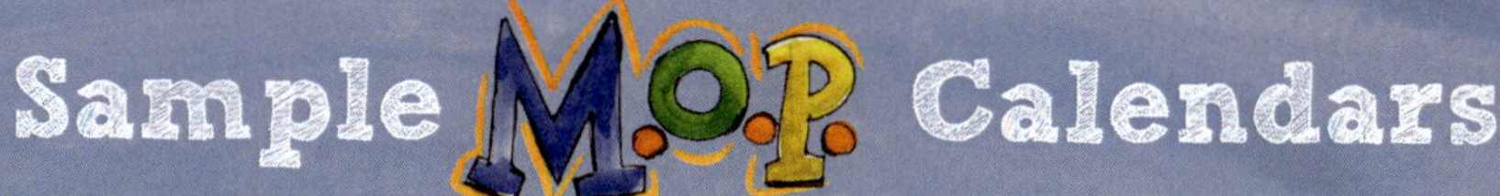

Sample #1

This child began **M.O.P.** with daily bedwetting, pee accidents, and urgency.

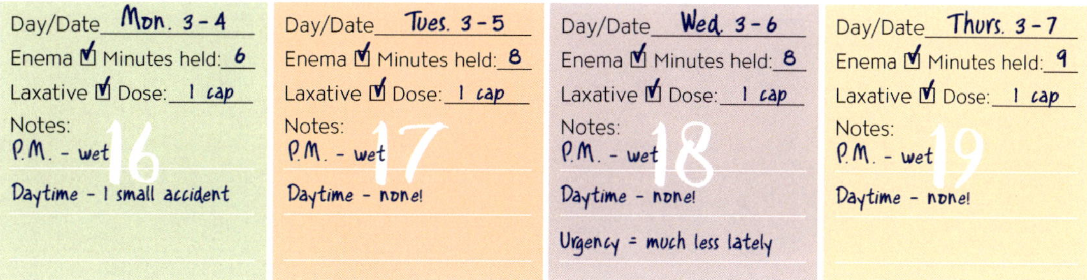

Day/Date Mon. 3-4	Day/Date Tues. 3-5	Day/Date Wed. 3-6	Day/Date Thurs. 3-7
Enema ☑ Minutes held: 6	Enema ☑ Minutes held: 8	Enema ☑ Minutes held: 8	Enema ☑ Minutes held: 9
Laxative ☑ Dose: 1 cap	Laxative ☑ Dose: 1 cap	Laxative ☑ Dose: 1 cap	Laxative ☑ Dose: 1 cap
Notes: 16	Notes: 17	Notes: 18	Notes: 19
P.M. - wet	P.M. - wet	P.M. - wet	P.M. - wet
Daytime - 1 small accident	Daytime - none!	Daytime - none!	Daytime - none!
		Urgency = much less lately	

Sample #2

This child began **M.O.P.** with bedwetting plus occasional pee and poop accidents.

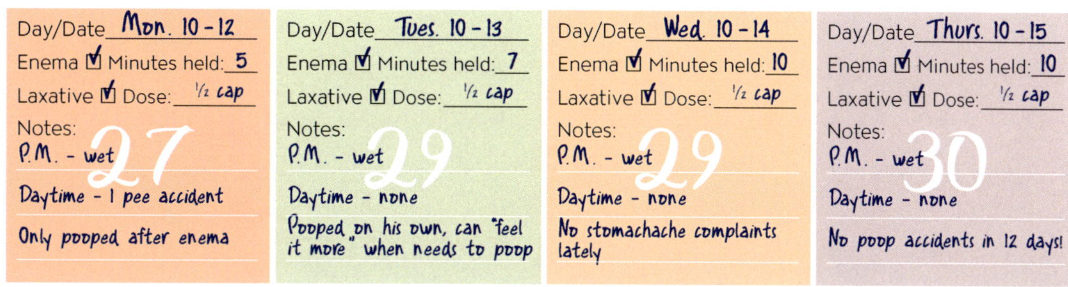

Day/Date Mon. 10-12	Day/Date Tues. 10-13	Day/Date Wed. 10-14	Day/Date Thurs. 10-15
Enema ☑ Minutes held: 5	Enema ☑ Minutes held: 7	Enema ☑ Minutes held: 10	Enema ☑ Minutes held: 10
Laxative ☑ Dose: ½ cap	Laxative ☑ Dose: ½ cap	Laxative ☑ Dose: ½ cap	Laxative ☑ Dose: ½ cap
Notes: 27	Notes: 29	Notes: 29	Notes: 30
P.M. - wet	P.M. - wet	P.M. - wet	P.M. - wet
Daytime - 1 pee accident	Daytime - none	Daytime - none	Daytime - none
Only pooped after enema	Pooped on his own, can "feel it more" when needs to poop	No stomachache complaints lately	No poop accidents in 12 days!

Assessing Your Child's Poop

How's Your Poop?
Yay!
Healthy Poop
Smooth mushy snakes
mushy blobs
soft-serve ice cream
Oh No!
Clogged Colon
rabbit pellets
big ol' logs
thick & bumpy sausage
© Cristina Acosta

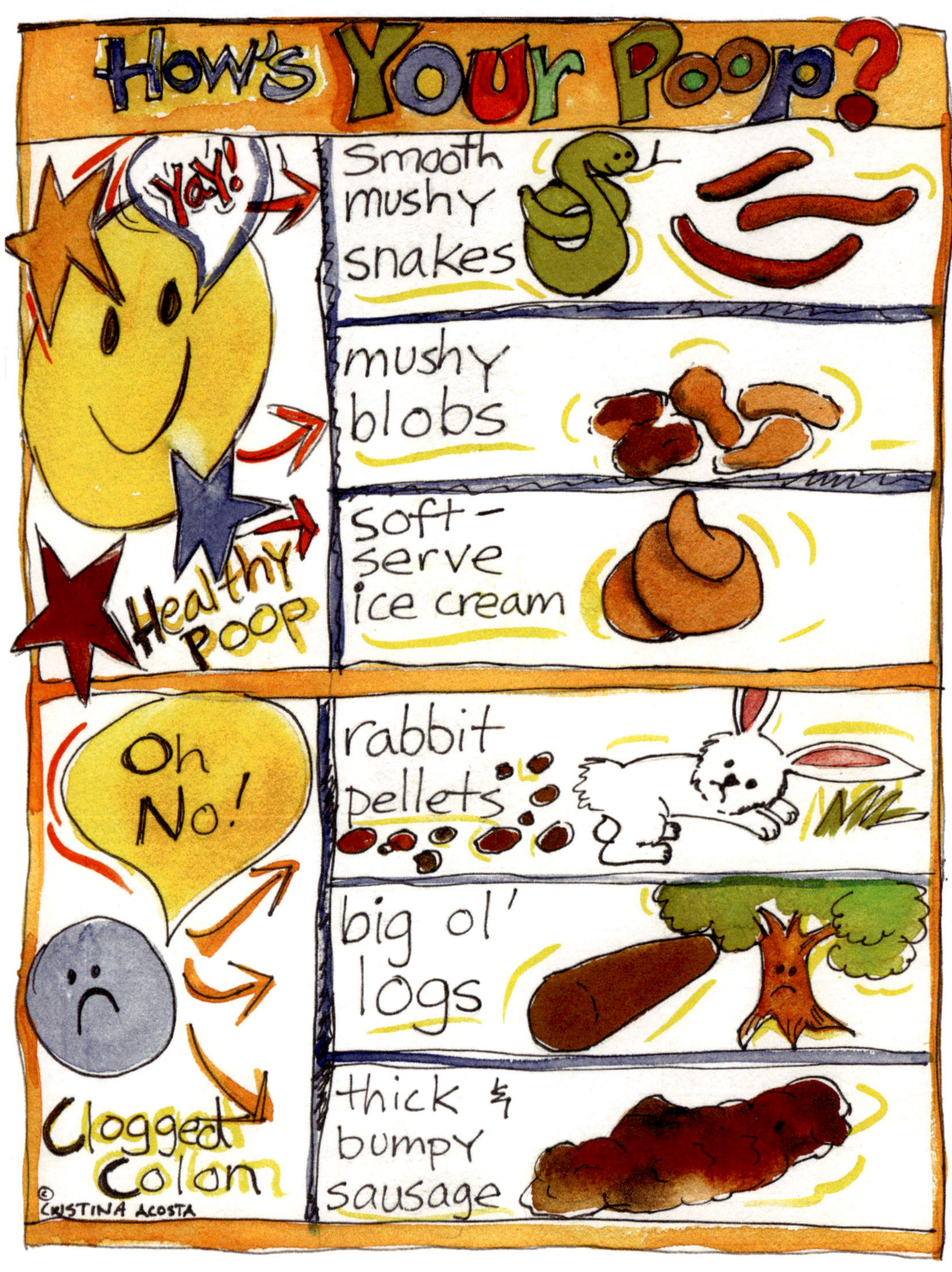

PART 6

RESOLVING THE TOUGHEST CASES:

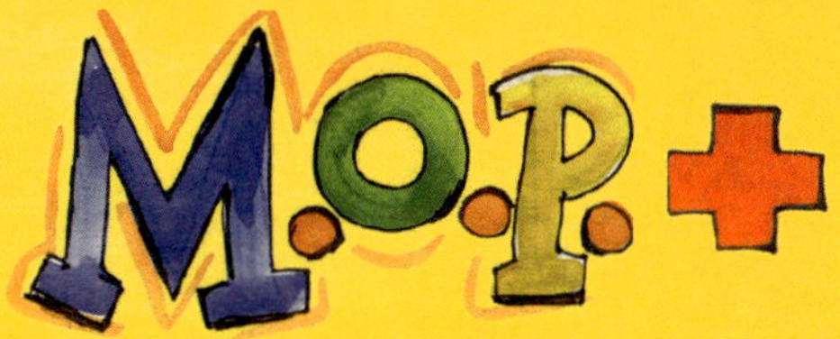

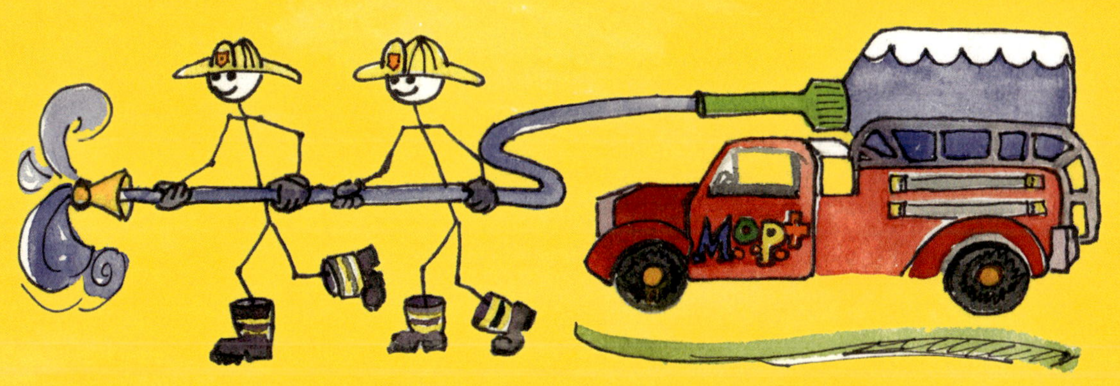

PART 6:

RESOLVING THE TOUGHEST CASES: M.O.P.+

I know it seems impossible that a child could still be having accidents after 30 consecutive days of enemas, but it happens. And when it does, I feel terrible, especially because these families typically have suffered the longest.

When a child's symptoms have not improved after a month or when improvement is negligible, it almost always means that the child's rectum is still clogged. An X-ray can tell you for sure. Parents are often blown away when an X-ray shows their child still has a massive rectal clog after a month of daily enemas.

I suggest you stay the course with **M.O.P.** if your child makes some progress — for example, if bedwetting persists but daytime accidents are diminishing. But if you observe no progress at all, it's time to move on.

The good news: There's always something else to try. Plan B is **M.O.P.+**, which is actually an array of options. Yes, there are Plans C and D, too, described in this section. Be prepared for a fair amount of trial and error. There's no way to predict which specific regimen will work for your child.

What is M.O.P.+?

M.O.P.+ is the same regimen as **M.O.P.**, with two differences:

1.) You use large-volume enemas instead of pediatric enemas. Large-volume enemas hold far more solution (300 to 600 cc) than pediatric enemas (66 cc) or even adult storebought enemas (about 130 cc). The larger volume stimulates the colon more aggressively to flush out crusty stool.

You can't buy these enemas ready-made, so **M.O.P.+** takes more work. The tradeoff: these enemas more effectively clean out a stubbornly mucked-up, rectum. I know: "large-volume enema" sounds scary, like you'll be spraying a fire hose up your child's bottom. In reality, these enemas are gentle. My patients, relieved there's a next strategy to try, tend to get on board quickly.

2.) You (possibly) add a stimulant to the saline solution. Store-bought pediatric enema solution typically contains saline plus phosphate, an electrolyte that draws water into the colon. Large-volume solution contains saline alone or saline plus one or more liquid stimulants, such as glycerin or castile soap. These liquids draw extra fluid into the colon, stimulating contractions and lubricating stool. You can change the solution at any time. **For sure make a change after a week if your child's poop output doesn't increase; don't use the same solution for more than 30 days if you see no improvement in symptoms.**

M.O.P.+ Supply List

With **M.O.P.+**, you buy (and reuse) the enema components and purchase or make your own solution. While this is more trouble, it's also much less expensive.

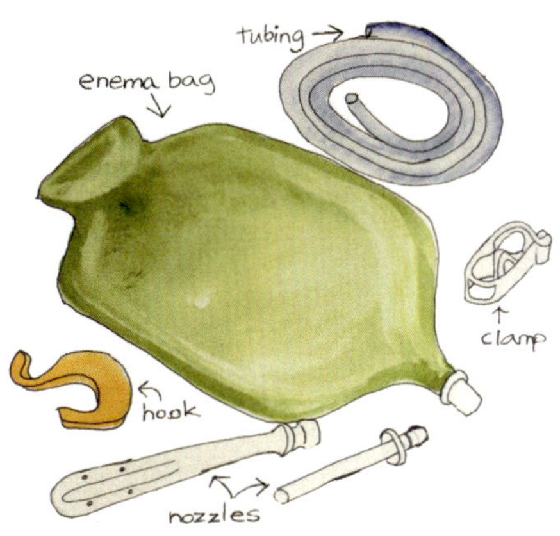

Reusable enema bag kits are available online.

Here's your shopping list.

You won't need all these items to begin.

Petrolum jelly Lubricant for the nozzle tip. Some parents report that their children prefer K-Y Jelly to Vaseline.

Enema bag plus accessories. Kits include enema bag, tubing, clamp, nozzles, hook, and tip. (Try Amazon, Walmart, and enemasupply.com.) The hook holds the bag, the bag holds the fluid, the long tubing sends the fluid down, and the nozzle enters the child's bottom. (For smaller children, use a child-sized tip. Search "flex tip enema junior nozzle.") The clamp turns the flow on and off. The Perfect Enema Bag Kit and the MABIS system are two good options. This video shows how to assemble the parts: youtube.com/watch?v=yXb9VSfX-WY

Solution. Here are the formulations we typically recommend in my practice.

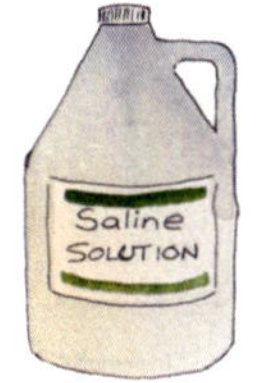

Saline: Buy saline solution online or at a pharmacy, or mix it yourself by adding 1 ½ teaspoons table salt to 1000 ml tap water. Measure the salt and water exactly so the sodium concentration is safe. Store extra solution at room temperature for later use. It's fine to use room-temperature water, though some children find warmer water (up to 100 degrees) more comfortable.
Ages 4 to 7: Start with 300 cc.
Ages 8+: Start with 600 cc.

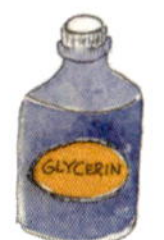

Glycerin: If saline enemas don't help, add 10 to 30 cc of glycerin — a thick, clear, sugar-based liquid — to the enema volume you're using. (5 cc is a teaspoon; 15 cc is a tablespoon.) A higher dose may be more effective but may also feel more uncomfortable to your child.

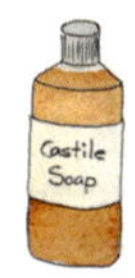

Liquid castile soap: If you're not making progress, add 10 to 30 cc of liquid castile soap, a plant-based soap, to the enema volume you are using. (Keep or drop the glycerin.) Or, you can use the same amount of Johnson's No More Tears Baby Shampoo. Yes, baby shampoo!

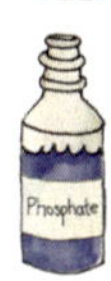

Fleet phosphate enemas: Still no progress? Add (to the glycerin and/or soap) ½ a pediatric Fleet or generic-brand enema if your child is age 3, a full pediatric phosphate enema in kids ages 4 to 10, and an adult phosphate enema in kids over 10.

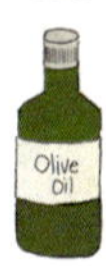

Olive oil and glycerin suppositories: These items do not go in the enema solution; see "Two more tricks in the bag," on page 44.

5 Steps to Giving a Large-Volume Enema

Giving a large-volume enema is not a whole lot different from giving a pediatric enema but may take some practice both for parent and child. I recommend administering the enema on the floor near the toilet. For many kids, watching a video on a phone or tablet is a welcome distraction.

Step 1 **Lubricate the tip of the tube, and show your child the enema bag and tube with lubricated tip.** Remind your child that while this may feel awkward or uncomfortable at first, kids report that it starts to feel routine after a few days.

Step 2 **Place a towel on the floor, and instruct your child to lie on his or her left side, knees bent.**

Step 3 **Gently insert the nozzle into the anus as high as possible.** You'll know you are in when you pass the point of resistance and when you squeeze and no liquid leaks back out. Encourage your child to take slow, deep breaths to help relax the sphincter. Tensing up can make the process uncomfortable. Some older children feel more relaxed if they hold the nozzle themselves.

Step 4 **Attach the hose to the enema bag, hold the bag about 2 feet above the floor, and begin the enema.** If the child complains of cramps, slow the flow by lowering the enema bag. It should take just a few minutes for the colon to fill.

Step 5 **When all the solution has entered the colon, remove the hose.** The child should aim to retain the fluid for at least 5 minutes (if possible), ideally for 10 minutes. The child should then sit on the toilet for 10 to 20 minutes. Clean the nozzle with soap and water or rubbing alcohol after each use.

"The large-volume enemas were a little tricky at first but have become very routine. In the early days, we had saline leaking out while we were trying to administer the enema, so we had to slow down the flow. Now we don't have any leaking, maybe because my son is better cleaned out."
– Mom of an 8-year-old boy

Two More Tricks in the Bag

If you're not getting anywhere with glycerin, castile soap, and/or phosphate, try the following two remedies, used with success by some families in our private Facebook group.

- **Add solid glycerin suppositories.** Remember, the goal is for the child to poop once a day in addition to pooping after the enema. For a child who is pooping only after the enema, it's reasonable to use a solid glycerin suppository in the morning to kickstart the colon until the child is pooping spontaneously once a day.
- **Inject 50 cc to 100 cc of olive oil before bed, and let it sit overnight.** Then, in the morning, begin the enema. The olive oil softens and lubricates the stool, so it empties more easily. Use an enema syringe (Universal Tube Cleanser is a good one) to measure and inject the olive oil. Do this right before bed, after your child has used the toilet for the last time. If the olive oil prompts your child to use the toilet one more time, that's OK, but the goal should be to hold in the olive oil for at least 20 minutes.

Insights into M.O.P.+

I'll be honest: I have much more experience with **M.O.P.** than I do with **M.O.P.+**. The vast majority of my clinic patients succeed with **M.O.P.**; only since I began sharing **M.O.P.** online did I discover that a substantial number of families need a more aggressive approach.

I'm guessing this is because the folks who find my website have children with the toughest cases. These parents have "tried everything" their doctor recommended, to no avail, and are still searching for answers. Most of their children are school aged and have been struggling with enuresis and/or encopresis for many years. At this point, pediatric enemas just won't do the job.

Many of these parents have joined our private Facebook group, where they share ideas, successes, and failures. I've found their comments and questions invaluable, and I learn from these parents every day.

M.O.P.+ is a work in progress and no doubt will be refined over time. But it's never going to be a cut-and-dried regimen. You have to keep tinkering with the various parts of the protocol until you find what works for your child. Below are some insights I've gleaned from families who have gone the **M.O.P.+** route. I'm grateful to the parents who have joined our Facebook group and have posted their experiences — both positive and negative — for others to learn from.

- **Wetting symptoms may worsen before they improve.** Right after starting **M.O.P.+**, some children experience more frequent or more severe wetting. Parents will write, "Suddenly, her pull-ups aren't just wet; they're soaked!" This can happen because the high volume of enema solution places even more pressure on the bladder nerves — which, of course, are already extremely aggravated from the severe constipation. Once the large-volume enemas start clearing out the clogged rectum, usually within a couple days, the situation will improve.
- **Some children feel nauseous when they start large-volume enemas.** A few even throw up. This happens for the same reason wetting symptoms can worsen: The colon is, temporarily, stretched even further. The GI tract is all connected, so the stretching down below sends waves upward, causing a more generalized bloating of the bowel. If this happens to your child, offer assurance that the nausea will soon subside.
- **Probiotics are not likely to help.** Probiotics, known as "good bacteria," can help maintain normal bacterial colonies in the colon, especially after an illness like viral diarrhea. However, despite lots of hype on the Internet, I have seen no compelling evidence to suggest they help alleviate chronic, severe constipation.

"I kept track of how much glycerin we added and how long my son was able to hold the enema. If his hold time was consistently short, I would cut back a bit on the glycerin. Once he started to consistently hold longer, I would slowly increase the dosage."
– Mom of boy on M.O.P.+

- **Make a change every 30 days.** As I've mentioned elsewhere, do not stick with a regimen that isn't working! It doesn't matter how many enemas you give your child; if the child's symptoms are not improving, the rectum is still clogged, and you need to move on. If you don't believe your child's rectum is clogged, get an X-ray. Parents will say, "My child has had a large-volume enema every single day for 4 months and is still wetting the bed! There's no way she can still be clogged." But we do an X-ray and guess what? The child is still clogged!

- **Tracking is essential.** You won't know when those 30 days are up unless you keep track. There are so many variables with **M.O.P.+**. Only by recording your child's specific regimen and symptoms can you figure out what is and isn't working.

Plan C: Beyond M.O.P.+

I know this is unthinkable, but if you've gotten this far, you may wonder: What if **M.O.P.+** doesn't work?

There is always another option to try. The next step is usually a Foley catheter, a tube for with a balloon at the end. The balloon creates a "seal" so the irrigation fluid doesn't leak back out, allowing you to fill the colon more fully. Ask your pediatrician or pediatric urologist about it.

When a Foley catheter isn't enough, I move on to the prescription Peristeen pump — basically an enema on steroids. It cleans out even the most stubbornly clogged children. If your pediatric GI doctor isn't familiar with it, contact me.

Recommended Progression for M.O.P.+
Saline Solution
First, try saline.
Then . . .
Add glycerin.
Then . . .
Glycerin
Castile Soap
Add castile soap.
Then . . .
Add phosphate. Then . . .
Phosphate
Olive Oil
Add overnight olive oil or morning suppositories. Then . . .
Try Foley catheter. Then . . .
Try Peristeen pump.

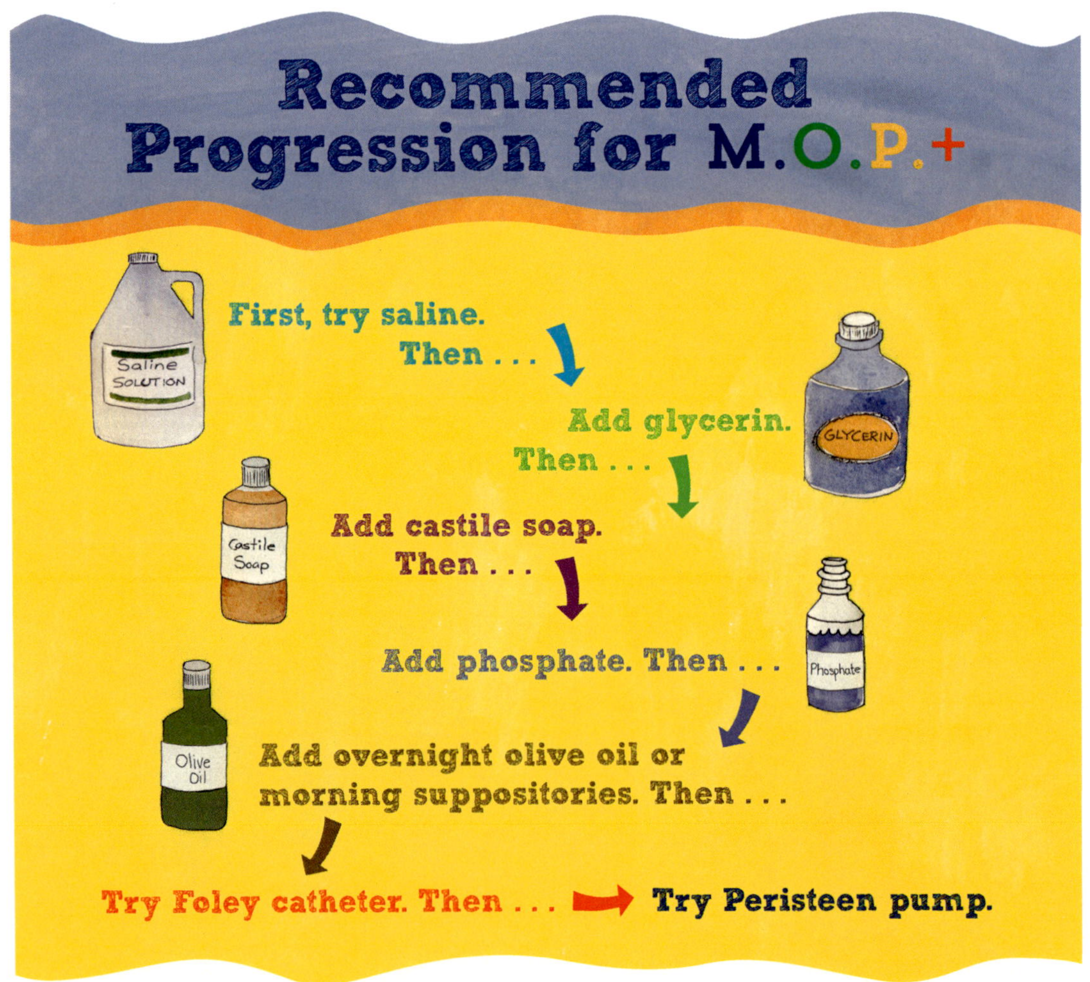

PART 7

PREVENTING A RELAPSE

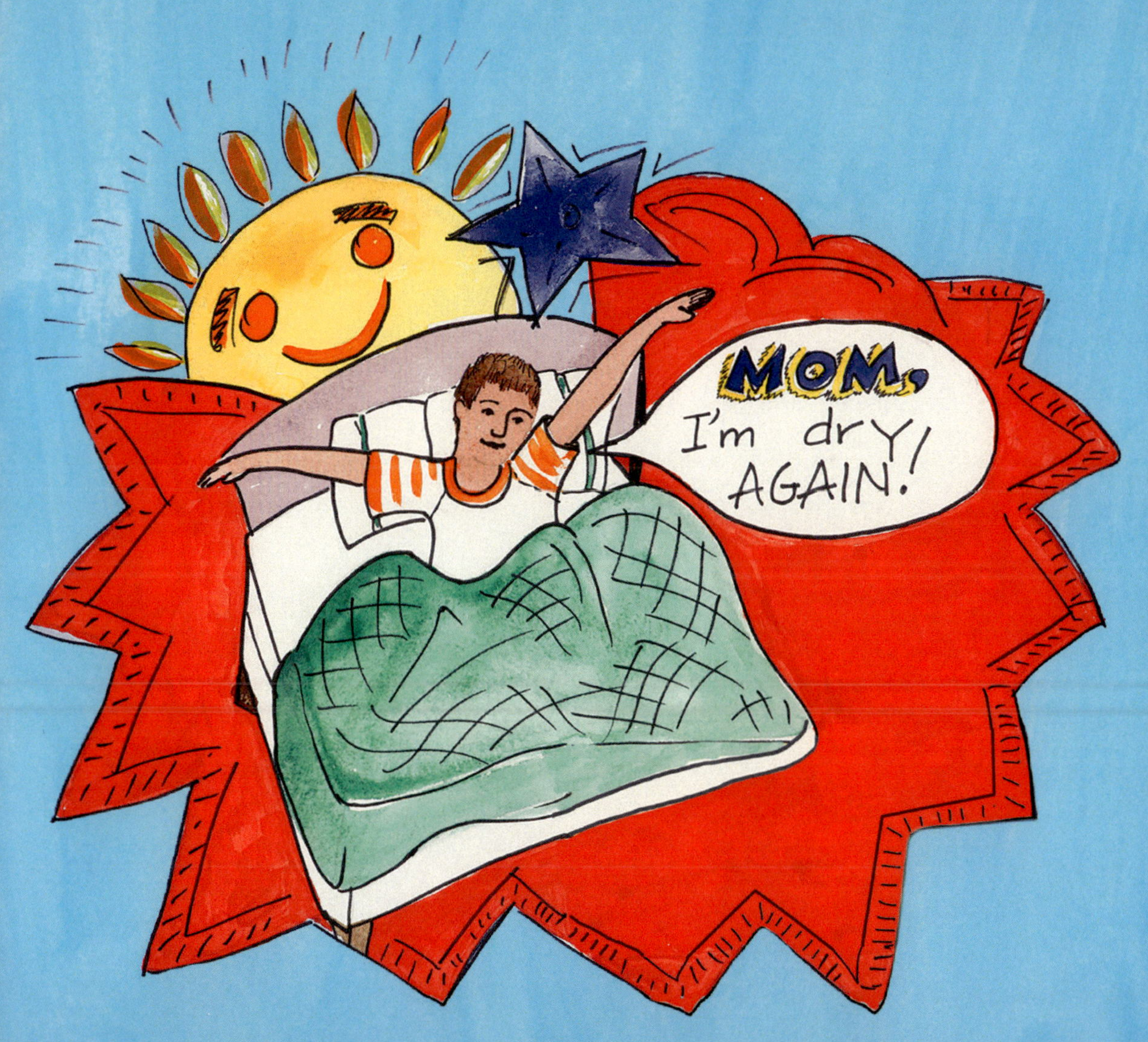

PART 7:
PREVENTING A RELAPSE

Once your child achieves dryness, you will surely never want to utter the word "enema" again!

And with luck and diligence, you won't have to. However, most kids who wet the bed or have accidents have been constipated for years and have developed habits that are deeply ingrained. Even when pooping is no longer painful, it's hard for kids to overcome their instinct to withhold poop and pee.

These kids are at high risk for a relapse, so the whole family needs to be vigilant to keep that from happening. To minimize the odds of a recurrence, a child should take these six steps:

Poop on a schedule.

Kids don't like to interrupt their lives to take a trip to the toilet, so they need to perceive pooping as a nonnegotiable part of their daily routine, like brushing their teeth. Of course, eventually they need to learn to go as soon as the urge hits, but at first, a schedule will help. After breakfast and after dinner are two great times to poop, as the urge to poop is generally strongest after eating, especially in the morning. In addition, your child should:

- **Sit on the toilet for a full five minutes.** Many kids pop off the toilet after 10 seconds, claiming they don't have to go. But if they just give it some time, they may empty a big pile of poop. Set a timer, and encourage your child to bring a favorite book or toy. Do this even if the child poops a small amount at first; more may be on the way!
- **Relax the sphincter.** When the abdominal muscles are tense, the pooping muscles are forced to relax, so encourage your child to blow into a balloon or into his hands while pooping.

Pee on a schedule.

Though a clogged rectum is the primary cause of bedwetting and accidents, holding pee contributes by causing the bladder wall to thicken and become hyperactive. Regular emptying is your child's friend! Constipated children should use the toilet right before bed, first thing in the morning, and about every two hours throughout the day.

If your child has a teacher who limits bathroom passes or rewards students for not using the bathroom during class time, explain that it's imperative for your child to have unrestricted bathroom access. Make this a priority! Print out *The K-12 Teacher's Fact Sheet on Childhood Toileting Troubles*, available on our website, and have your doctor write a note. If your doctor won't, I will!

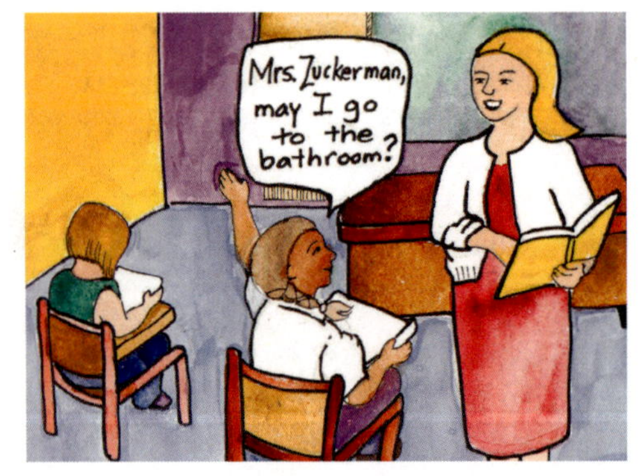

Explain to your child's teacher why your child needs unrestricted bathroom access.

Many kids don't want to "waste" recess or lunch period in the bathroom or are too embarrassed to raise their hand during class. Or, they just may forget to go because they habitually hold their pee. In all these cases, I recommend getting your child a watch that can be set to vibrate.

Eat "real food."

Nothing clogs up a child's insides like a diet of sugary cereals, goldfish crackers, chicken nuggets, and gummy bears! Switching to real food — you know, items your great-grandparents would have recognized as food, as opposed to the packaged, chemical-laden "products" that often pass for food in our culture — can make a dramatic difference in how your child poops and feels. There are loads of excellent websites to help. Two of the best are 100 Days of Real Food and Real Mom Nutrition.

Poop with a stool — for life.

Your child will probably always be prone to constipation, so pooping in the squatting position needs to be a lifelong habit. As your child grows, upgrade to a taller stool, and set an example by pooping with a stool yourself! All of us, regardless of age, should be pooping in a squat.

Drink plenty of fluids.

You'd be amazed at how little most kids drink! Stopping life to sip water is just not a habit for most kids. But it needs to be! Drinking fluids through the day will keep your child's bladder on a constant filling/emptying cycle. Drinking a few ounces every few hours, rather than guzzling a whole bottle at once, ensures the bladder doesn't fill too quickly or remain empty for too long. Rapid filling can cause bladder overactivity; a bladder is happiest when it's in a cycle of gradually filling and regularly emptying.

Invite your child to choose a fun water bottle to keep in the classroom and another to carry around outside of school.

Stay active.

Fewer than 10% of K-12 schools offer daily P.E., and most kids fall way short of the recommended 60 minutes of physical activity each day. Yet exercise is critical to keeping your child's insides humming along. Help your kids find fun activities that involve moving their bodies!

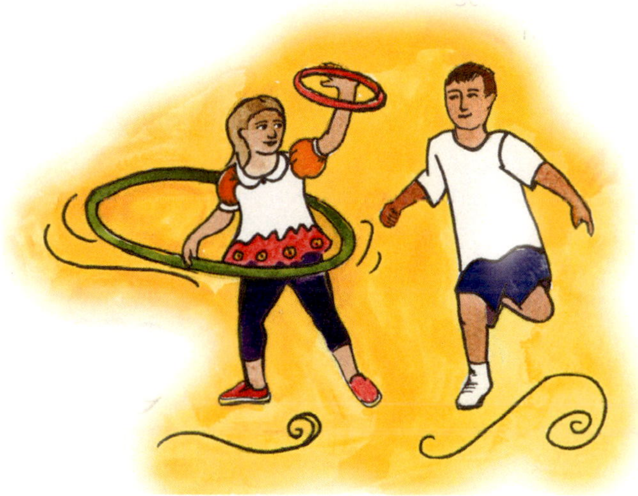

Exercise keeps the colon humming!

Families Love Our Children's Book

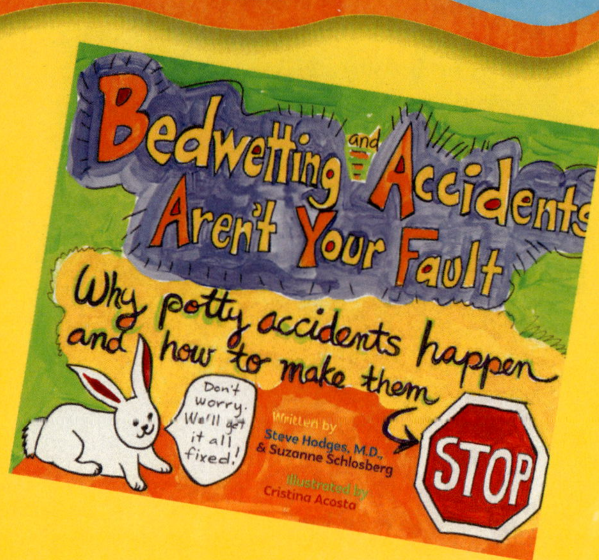

From Verified Amazon Purchasers
4.7 out of 5 stars!

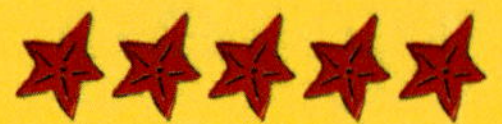

Excellent Explanation!

My child was totally on board with the treatments after reading the book.

Great Cliff's Notes

Our son likes this book and wants to read it every day, often while he's on the toilet :)

We LOVED this book

I bought this for my kids to read and learn, but I ended up learning and being entertained at the same time.

Fantastic book

Reading this picture book really helped our daughter be calm and prepared for the idea of getting an enema.

I wish I had known about this book 4 years ago!

The illustrations and writing style are very kid-friendly and even made my son laugh about a topic that he normally avoids if at all possible.

Great for kids of all ages!

I read this to my 5- and 7-year-old. Its fun, breezy style helps the topic feel comfortable and humorous.

Dr. Pooper is a ROCKSTAR!!!

When my son didn't want to go use the bathroom, I'd remind him, "What does Dr. Pooper want you to do every day?" and that would convince him to give it a try!

From Verified Amazon Purchasers
4.9 out of 5 stars!

A Deeper Dive Into The M.O.P. Story

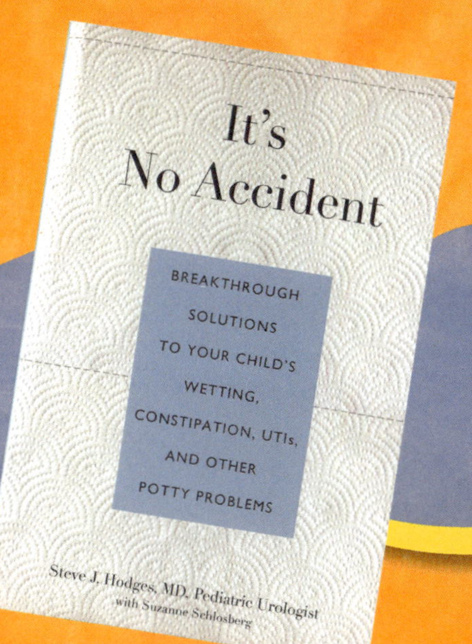

Should be mandatory for all pediatricians

My son would wake up and apologize for being wet. It broke my heart. The doctor pretty much told my son it was his fault. This book MADE SENSE, unlike the explanations from my pediatrician.

This is her one chance at a happy childhood

A life changer for our 5-year-old daughter. Only wish we'd found it sooner.

A must read

Two pediatricians, a GI specialist, and a urologist were not able to help our son. Finally, I found this book and now my son is dry.

It's like they studied my daughter

I wish I had access to this book 10 years ago! So many heartaches and embarrassments could have been avoided.

This book is brilliant

I read several books by so-called experts, but after I read this one, I dropped the rest in a parking-lot book drop.

Mind blown!

I was so tired of hearing "He'll grow out of it." After reading this book, it all made sense.

Highly recommended

This book solved our scream, pull-your-hair-out problems. Life changing!

Made in the USA
Middletown, DE
09 June 2018